AF480792

PERSEVERING

A Complete Guide to Applications, Schools, and Work Opportunities for Foreign-Trained Dentists in the United States

Sampada Deshpande, DDS

Cover image photo by Front Range Ride Guides

ISBN: 979-8-9851301-0-2 (Hardcover)

ISBN: 979-8-9851301-1-9 (Ebook)

To mom,
who always believed in me, even when I did not.

CONTENTS

FOREWORD

As a practice owner, I have interviewed several dental assistants and front desk personnel as potential candidates. Many times, I encountered foreign-trained dentists who were either in the pro-cess of applying to US dental schools or those who had given up on becoming a dentist in the United States. Many mentioned that the process for a foreign-trained dentist to become an American dentist remained challenging, either due to financial reasons or the time commitment required. It is truly regrettable that some of these bright individuals did not get to fulfill their dreams or contribute their talents after spending years of education and practice in their home country.

Without a doubt, it is a long journey to become a dentist, and if you are foreign trained, the process is lengthier and more complicated. Dr. Sampada Deshpande, who moved from the Middle East to the West Coast and now lives in the San Francisco Bay Area, came on top as a winner in this process. She received American Dental Association's prestigious "10 under 10" Award, having lived in the US for fewer than 10 years. She decided to share her experiences in her first book, *Persevering,* with the rest of the world: she has laid out the process of school applications program by program; compiled others' experiences in this book; and stressed not only on the academic aspects of the preparation but also the right mindset that would serve to prepare oneself as an ideal candidate. You can be in any part of the world and still be able to gain insight on how to become a dentist in the US and Canada by reading this book.

As the book title suggests, *Persevering* requires persistent hard work over time. *Persevering* is a much-needed handbook with practical advice and up-to -date information for foreign-trained dentists, from application requirements to interviews to life in dental school and eventually to life after dental school. This book encompasses every element needed for a foreign-trained dentist to succeed in America and Canada.

I applaud Dr. Sampada Deshpande for her efforts in writing this much-needed book for our dental profession, and I would recommend this book to every foreign-trained dentist who is con-sidering becoming a dentist in the US and Canada. "Perseverance is not a long race; it is many short races one after the other", said Walter Elliot. *Persevering* signifies the constant motion of these short races that would only lead to success in time.

—Cathy Hung, DDS, FAAOMS, CLC
Author of *Pulling Wisdom and Behind Her Scalpel*

INTRODUCTION

International dentists who plan to move to the US are curious to know the different pathways for foreign-trained dentists to pursue their dental education or practice dentistry in the US. This book is sure to answer most of the questions they may have in that journey.

"The key to success is action and the essential in action is Perseverance" Dr. Sampada has brought this out in her book through the thoughtfully written twelve chapters beginning with the chapter on Staying True to Your "Why". It is very important to understand your 'why' and to work towards it with passion.

"If a window of opportunity appears, don't pull down the shade." Dr. Sampada has emphasized this in Chapter 2, "Becoming the ideal candidate."

"You have to learn the rules of the game. And then, you have to play better than anyone else". It is essential to know the requirements of the various dental schools before you apply and this is well explained in Chapter 3. The information pertaining to 40 American universities offering dental programs is comprehensive.

Chapter 4 speaks of ways to boost your CV for strengthening your candidature and stresses on the fact that it's never too early to start.

Chapter 5 on bench tests - a skills evaluation to test practical and clinical knowledge conducted by admission committees of universities, gives an insight into the author's personal experience and that of others.

Chapter 6 gives advice on preparing for the personal interview. Being able to choose the right dental school is very important and so is liking what you have chosen. This is well featured in Chapter 7 and 8.

Determining how to practice dentistry is a different question than just recognizing what kind of dentistry you want to practice. Chapter 9 throws light on different options available after completion of dental school.

An international dentist could join an accredited post-graduate program and apply for a license thereafter instead of going back to school for an Advanced Standing program like Dr. Sampada did. This is not an option for all states however and is a route filled with many challenges, and specifications. Chapter 10 enlightens the reader about such residency programs for international dentists.

Like in the US, dentistry in Canada is also highly regulated. Chapter 11 guides the international candidate for an effective transition in Canada.

The last chapter is a collection of final thoughts and advice gathered from dentists and students interviewed for the book and provides the reader with further mentorship.

"Some people want it to happen, some wish it would happen, others make it happen", Dr. Sampada Deshpande, the author of Persevering, belongs to the third category. I have seen her as an undergraduate dental student from 2008 to 2013 and today I am very happy and proud that she has successfully paved her way to becoming a dentist in the United States of America. Her concerted efforts in compiling a book for foreign trained dentists are highly appreciable and I am very sure that this handbook will be of great help to anyone wanting to become a dentist in the US.

—Dr. Keerthilatha M. Pai, Dean, Manipal
College of Dental Sciences, Manipal University

PREFACE

Hi,

I am a general dentist based in the San Francisco Bay Area. A few years after graduating from dental school at Manipal University, India, I began my two-year Advanced Standing DDS program at the University of Washington in Seattle, Washington, in the year 2016.

Getting licensed to practice in the United States, after having been through dental school in another country, can take you many years. Yes, years! There are also various ways to go about it. Many dentists choose not to go through what I did, which is the Advanced Standing program, a 2-3 year long, highly competitive and expensive process, to get their license.

Why are you holding this book?
You have already combed through several resources readily avail-able and still find yourself confused about where to begin. Or you are currently in dental school and are interested to know what it takes to begin practicing as a fully licensed dentist in America. Or perhaps, you are looking for mentorship from someone who has been through the process you are about to embark on.

Whatever the situation, know that you are in the right place. I get asked about my journey as a foreign-trained dentist about once a week. There are things I know now about the process that I wish I knew then. I have realized over the years that what is missing from resources available on the internet is students' personal experiences and specific advice that would give candidates a fighting chance.

Therefore, I decided to compile a book about my experiences and those of other colleagues, detailing pitfalls to avoid and imparting advice on developing a competitive edge.

Why did it take me three cycles to get into an American dental school? Is that too long a time or too short?

I graduated from Manipal University in India thinking I'm exactly the kind of candidate that most dental schools in the US are look-ing for. Driven and motivated, I had been President of the Student Council, had hundreds of volunteering hours, received an award for community service, and high academic scores. Many success-ful students I knew at the time had gotten into DDS pro-grams within their first cycle. I assumed it would be the same for me.

Most dentists are naturally introverted and don't feel com-fortable asking others for help. This is where we fail collec-tively. Many times, it is the ego that stops us from addressing our own shortcomings; other times, it is a lack of knowledge. In my case, it was both. It wasn't until a year and a half into the process that I decided to ask a dear friend for feedback. Up until then, I didn't even know I needed feedback.

Think of this book as a friend who is gently prodding you to reevaluate your application. Advice in this book has been compiled with the help of several foreign- trained dentists like yourself, some of them having been through a string of rejections and who are now in their dream job, practice, or city. Consider their recommendations as personal feedback, and work relentlessly towards your goals.

This is a book tailored with advice for those applying to a DDS program in the United States. I've also added information about opportunities post-graduation and a bonus chapter on finding work in Canada. Although we interviewed several people who did things differently, our main audience is a foreign-trained dentist (FTD) looking at settling down in the States after completing a traditional two- or three-year-long Advanced Standing program.

Before you jump in, here's a reminder: You are not alone. You got this!

1

STAYING TRUE TO YOUR "WHY"

Several foreign-trained dentists, while in reputable inter-national programs across the country, have no idea what they want to do after graduation. What happened to the big goals they put on their statement of purpose? Many graduates follow what everyone else is doing and find themselves in a job—also known as an associateship—that does not help them meet their professional or personal goals. They end up dispirited, disappointed, and bored.

One of those people was me.

What I found missing early in my career after graduation was the inability to stay true to my "why." Therefore, I highly recommend reading the book *Find your Why* by Simon Sinek. Reconnecting with your why will help you identify your five-and ten-year plans and inspire you to take the necessary steps to make your dreams come true.

For example, one of the breakthroughs I had after reading the book was realizing my passion for working with children with special needs. Almost a year later, I left my associateship at a big corporate dental office and enrolled in a government-funded Leadership and Education in Neurodevelopmental Disabilities (LEND) program at the University of Washington. The program helped lay the foundation for my vision of improving access to care for people with neurodevelopmental disabilities.

Having a why and working towards your passion should start before applying to dental schools. Many people from around the world have the false idea that practicing dentistry in the US will give them a better life. Although you can draw a decent income and a good lifestyle, finding a job, a practice to acquire, and having the right immigration status are far more complicated issues here in America than anywhere else. That, coupled with rising tuition and a higher cost of living, causes several foreign-trained dentists to take out big loans.

Is the effort worth it?
Yes, but only if it aligns with your why.

Maybe your ''why" is to do a residency and specialize in a niche field of dentistry. You may not always need to complete a traditional DDS program to make that happen. See Chapter 10 to read about my colleague's journey doing just that.

Or maybe your ''why" is to have your own practice one day and be able to care for your community the way you always envi-sioned. In Chapter 9, you'll learn of my colleague's experience building his pediatric dental practice.

People take different pathways to living out their dreams. If one path does not work, you should have other ideas to imple-ment. This book provides you with those ideas, so keep reading.

2

BECOMING THE IDEAL CANDIDATE

One of the most common questions I hear is, "How do I improve my chances of getting accepted into a US den-tal school?" This section details a list of extracurricular activities you can get involved in at any stage of your career to help you become a well-rounded candidate.

This chapter deliberately does not talk about clinical require-ments and academic scores from your previous dental school. Here is why; clinical requirements and academic scores vary greatly based on which country you graduated from. Your clinical skill will be judged at a prospective school's bench exam-ination. A bench examination is what schools use to calibrate students com-ing from different countries, and often differ-ent disciplines too. For details on bench examinations, head to Chapter 5. Academic scores reflect a candidate's ability to thrive in a challenging and new environment. If you haven't fared well previously, how would you be able to keep up now?

However, contrary to popular notion, many successful can-didates have a less than average GPA (grade point average). You need more than just your academic scores to demonstrate your passion for dentistry, further education, and community engage-ment. While a 4.0 GPA does not hurt, one cannot assume that a good GPA by itself will be sufficient in being successful. At a 3.8 GPA, it certainly was not in my case.

What I know now is that schools are not looking for book-smart students. They are looking for well-rounded doctors who will make a difference in their communities. So, even if you have a low GPA, you can still make it. And rock your interview.

FINDING A CAUSE

Find a cause close to your heart, and volunteer at a center that supports that cause. It doesn't have to be dentistry- related; it need not even be in healthcare. It only must be a cause you believe in.

For example, one of my favorite places to volunteer as a dental student at Manipal University was *Asare-* a center for children and young adults with developmental disabilities. This center offered recreational activities and vocational training to its students. Often, I would spend my Sunday mornings tak-ing students for walks, exercising with them, and listening to music. These activities never felt like work. They were just a lot of fun! These memories later helped me understand what patient interactions I valued the most in my career and what my dream practice should be like.

Fast-forward to my year of internship when I became president of the Student Council. When our council thought of organizing a community dental clinic benefiting the children and young adults at Asare, we received a lot of encouragement from our dental school faculty. We organized four such successful dental clinics that year alone. Students at the center received much-needed dental exams, cleanings, and fillings. More involved treatments were referred to the dental school. On the other hand, dental students were able to hone their interpersonal and leadership skills and learn how to build rapport with patients. It was a very fulfilling experience.

Ultimately, this opportunity became a major talking point at Advanced Standing interviews. I found that faculty enjoy speaking to students who go out of their way to connect the dots and initiate a project that means something to them.

Ask yourself: What am I passionate about? What can I ini-tiate on someone else's behalf? How involved am I in my local community?

SAY YES!

Say yes to opportunities that come your way. While at Manipal University, my senior in dental school started a non-profit called the Oral Cancer Organization (OCO). When he asked for help in conducting oral cancer screening clinics for the population in and around Manipal, I was quick to say yes.

Oral cancer is the most common type of cancer observed in the South Asian population. This is because of the high preva-lence of tobacco chewers. As dental students, we would often see advanced cases of cancer amongst our patients.

Together, our small team at the OCO created and distributed educational pamphlets and posters within our local community. We also conducted clinics offering cancer screening to employees of the transportation department in our university. Although not originally the intention, saying yes to the opportunity opened doors to an academic paper for board members to work on together as a team. This paper ultimately went on my resume and became a fond memory of collaboration and teamwork.

STUDENT GOVERNMENT

Being in student government, at any position, teaches you import-ant skills in people management, communication, and leadership. As a member of student government, you will find several oppor-tunities simply because you are in a position of responsibility. People will often think of involving you first because it lends credibility to their projects. Therefore, it is crucial to be involved in organized dentistry and student government as much as possible.

Being involved in a ton of projects is not easy. It requires hard work, long nights, and managing time well. However, with the right mindset, you will thrive in such a dynamic environment. After a rigorous selection process, I was chosen to be a member of a team to go to Ladakh, India, to offer comprehensive dental care to children and adults with reduced access to dental services. This project, *Amchi*, (Amchi is a term in Marathi that means ours) was hosted by my school in collaboration with the European Dental Student Association (EDSA). This became an opportunity for me to meet dental students from different countries and understand how dentistry is practiced elsewhere.

My role in this endeavor was to collect funding from sponsors, set up inventory, and organize clinics once we were in Ladakh. It was tough work, but it became my initial foray into running a small business. I learned early on how to allocate expenses on a profit and loss statement, perform basic accounting, and maintain a marketing budget. This work is the reason I became interested in the business side of dentistry. Several years later, I started an educational nonprofit called New Dentist Business Club in the US, utilizing what I learned first in *Amchi*.

Travel For Conferences

Participate in national conferences and be active in presenting papers or posters while in school. Many schools offer you a stipend for representing your university at a national conference. Make use of this opportunity and meet dental students and faculty from all over the country. Placing first or second in a paper pre-sentation is not the crucial aspect here. Watching others present and looking at a diverse set of academic papers will open your mind to new ideas. You may find yourself thinking critically about different aspects of dentistry and be influenced to work on a new academic paper later.

BUILD RELATIONSHIPS

Work on building genuine relationships with your colleagues and the faculty at your dental school. They are the same people who will write you a letter of recommendation, proofread your state-ment of purpose, or give advice about getting into an Advanced Standing program. You want someone deeply invested in your professional success to write a glowing letter of recommendation for you.

Dhara Patel, a current D3 (third year dental student) at the International DDS program at the University of Washington, has the following advice:

Begin working on letters of recommendation (LOR) as soon as possible. All LOR's are valid only for six months, but give your professors enough time to write something personal about you. One of the reasons I wasn't invited to the University of California San Francisco (UCSF) was because a professor wrote a very generic letter of recommendation for me. I was given this feedback by the UCSF program counselor when I called and asked about what changes I can make to my application next time.

Your application gets limited facetime when it reaches a school. Letters of recommendation and the statement of purpose are often the first things that any faculty member reads. Make them count. And know that it all starts with building authentic relationships with your colleagues and professors first.

NETWORKING

Spend time working with the community outside of your den-tal school; become friends with students in other disciplines, if you can. We often fail to realize that students in other disci-plines will be our colleagues soon. We can learn a lot from them. Interdisciplinary learning can be critical in problem-solving on a grand scale.

Many of my friends in Manipal University participated in entrepreneur competitions where they worked with students from different schools to put forth business ideas that could potentially change our respective industries. Even if you don't win at such competitions, the experience itself is amazing. It provides a plat-form to improve your public speaking skills while also building lifelong friendships.

Well-Rounded Candidates

It is imperative to work on developing a well-rounded person-ality and getting into the mindset of a positive, growth-minded individual.

We don't need more book-smart doctors around the world. We need compassionate people (who happen to be doctors) who will work hard for the betterment of the community. We need people who will inspire and motivate staff and patients, be involved in academia, and maintain a suitable work-life balance.

You don't have to aspire to be everything. Be a few things and do them very well. Read books, travel, and remember to laugh and enjoy yourself with your friends and family.

This is a marathon, not a sprint. Take care of yourself, carving out plenty of time for sleep and relaxation. If you do not have fun every minute of the day, will it even be worth it in the end?

Study Material, Timing, And Application Materials

Use your fourth year and internship to collect all study mate-rials and begin preparing for the INBDE (Integrated National Board Dental Examination) and TOEFL (Test of English as a Foreign Language). Results of the TOEFL are valid for only two years, so it may be best to take the test as late as possible. Use most of your internship year to focus on your boards, practice with past papers, and build a study group with other students. Remember that in the US, you are tested on full-body anatomy, unlike what we may learn in other countries. Keep that in mind when preparing. You will need enough time if you want to pass on your first attempt.

Dhara Patel has some advice on time management too:

During my internship, I had my grades converted with ECE (Educational Credential Evaluators) and WES (World Education Services). I'd recommend getting this done as soon as possible and ideally before you leave your home country. For example, it gets very difficult to get sealed transcripts later in the process. I did a master's degree in public health (MPH) program at St. John's University in NYC after graduating from dental school in India. My classes were only in the evening, so I would spend my mornings preparing for the NBDE parts I and II and studying for TOEFL.

Side Note: ECE and WES are two North American institutions that convert a foreign dental school tran-script to an American standard grade point average or GPA. Most dental schools in America accept transcripts from either or both. The INBDE, prior to 2020, used to be taken in 2 separate exams - NBDE part I and NBDE part II. At the time of this writing, most schools now also accept scores of the INBDE.

Interested in learning more about MPH? Visit Chapter 4 to read about gap years.

RESEARCH PAPERS

Involve yourself in research papers early. Speak to faculty in your school who have published papers. Ask them what they are working on and tell them you are interested in helping. It is okay to tell them you are working on building your resume and are willing to put in several hours to make your work count as an author.

Nayanika Sanga DDS, a general dentist based in British Columbia, Canada and a graduate of the University of Michigan advanced standing program, says, "I had the opportunity to present a research paper at an annual symposium while in my MPH program. I ended up getting second place in this competition. A lot of interviewers at Advanced Standing programs were interested in my research paper, and I was able to use the experience to illustrate my passion for dentistry effectively."

Research papers make a big difference to your resume. Professors are always looking for help in data collection, so many will be happy to get help. On the other hand, if you have ideas of your own, talk to your favorite faculty member and make that happen for yourself.

Side Note: It is acceptable to put research work on your resume alongside comments such as 'pending publication' or 'at proofreading stage' to let the admissions committee know what you are working on even if it is not published in a journal yet. Remember to be honest about the status of your research work, it is not okay to embellish.

3

SCHOOL REQUIREMENTS

S chools have been listed here in alphabetical order. We do not endorse any ranking system; all schools are unique and special in their own ways.

Before you dive in, here is a recommended timeline for com-pleting prerequisites, preparing for bench tests, and applying to schools.

American schools run either on a semester system or a quarter system. Semester systems divide the academic year into two main parts, whereas the quarter system separates it into four. Most dental schools run on a quarter system, so while explain-ing prerequisites, we will use the following example: assume an applicant is preparing to join school in the Fall quarter of 2025.

1. Centralized Application for Advanced Placement of International Dentists or <u>CAAPID</u> application cycle begins in March of the preceding year. So, for advanced standing programs that begin in the Fall quarter of 2025, the application cycle usually runs from March 2024 to Feb 2025.

2. Although the application cycle runs for 11 months, most schools accept applications only for two to three of those months. For example, most schools in California would accept applications until June 2024 only. You must keep in mind the school deadline, and not necessarily the CAAPID deadline, or you might miss out.

3. Many schools are on rolling -admissions. This means that those students who put in a completed application earlier on will have more chances to get an interview. Apply in March 2024, within a week or as soon as the cycle opens.

PRO TIP: It doesn't matter which school is on rolling admissions and which one isn't. In my third (and thankfully, final) cycle of applications, I had already learned my lesson and applied to every single school on my list within a week of the CAAPID application cycle opening. I got five interviews that year. Coincidence? Not at all. Apply early.

4. Complete the <u>INBDE</u> (as of this writing, NBDE Part 1 has been discontinued, and Part II will be discontinued in August 2022) before anything else. This means your exam should have been completed in early- to mid -2023, so you have enough time to focus on application requirements prior to submitting paperwork in March of 2024.

5. TOEFL scores typically last for two years only. Try to give this exam as late as possible so it remains valid for longer. This protects you against taking the exam again if you must apply for the following cycle. The ideal timing would be January 2024.

6. Some schools give you only two weeks to prepare for an interview (e.g., University of Washington), one month (e.g., Pacific), whereas others give you two to three months (e.g., University of Buffalo). Anticipating the interview and preparing for it months in advance is *key*. Do not wait to get an invite. If you do that, you will already be late and wasting the opportunity to interview.

PRO TIP: Attend a professional 10- to 15-day course at a test-ing center like Duggan Institute, right after you have finished the INBDE in mid-2023. This will give you at least six to nine months of preparation time at home. You will be extremely confident and well prepared when it comes time to interview.

You will crush it.

Learn from my failures. I began preparing only a month before my bench exam at Colorado in 2014. I was rejected. I realized at the interview how much more prepared everyone else was.

Learn from my wins. I happened to be at the Duggan Institute on August 10, 2015, when I got the interview invitation for the University of Washington (UW) for Aug 27–29. This was my second time practicing at the Institute. Each time I had spent more than a month practicing on mannequins and getting my work critiqued by Dr. Duggan. Pure coincidence that I received an invite 10 days prior to the interview at UW. I couldn't have asked for a better situation because at that very moment, I felt supremely confident. I went for the bench exam well prepared. The rest is history.

Study Material

Although everyone you meet will recommend different books and study material, here are a few of the courses and books that are being personally recommended by the author and contributors of this book.

TOEFL: Barron's with DVD, ibt practice papers

INBDE or parts 1 and 2: past ASDA (American Student Dental Association) test papers, Dental Decks

Individual School Breakdown

This is the part you have all been waiting for. There are just a couple of pointers before you dive in.

Please note that school requirements, facilities, and dead-lines change, and the most updated information will always be available on the school website. Listed in the following pages are details based on interviews with current students, graduates, and faculty as of Spring 2021. Many of the interviews have been left anonymous on purpose and are therefore in quotation marks.

Every effort was made to create a listing that is as compre-hensive as possible. However, not every school was able to give the author enough details. Those schools, understandably, have shorter descriptions. This in no part indicates anything negative about the school.

Forty schools have been mentioned below. In the coming years there may be more programs getting added. For an update, please go to the American Dental Association website for a full list of all schools accepting foreign-trained dentists, that either participate in CAAPID or not.

Finally, here are some clarifications. The term 'integration' in the following context indicates that the cohort of FTDs (Foreign-Trained Dentists) is in the same class, labs, or clinics as their domestic colleagues. The term 'Board' in the following pages refers to clinical boards that at the time of this writing, are required with graduation in order to receive a license to practice in a specific state of the US. Some schools are Board testing loca-tions and others are not. Lastly, in the US, instead of saying 'second years', we often refer to students as D2's. Similarly 'third year' students are referred to as D3's, so on and so forth. You will read that language in the following pages.

1. University of Alabama School of Dentistry

Integration	YES
Class size	16
City life and cost of living	"City life - Amazing. Birmingham is a small city with a big city feel. Lots of good food (especially BBQ!). This city has so many local breweries with signature local beers. I'm from the north, and I instantly fell in love with the southern hospitality. Cost of living - Birmingham downtown can be a little expensive. If you have friends and want to share an apartment, then it will be cheaper. Cheaper areas outside the city are in the suburbs, but for those who hate travelling to school (like me), living outside the city isn't an option because parking can be an issue!" Average cost of a 1 bed 1 bathroom (1b1b) apartment: $640/-
Length of program	30 months
What is special about the program?	"Ours is a very clinically heavy program. We probably have the highest number of patients in the country. Students graduate with a minimum requirement of 30-35 crowns! (I have not seen any other school with such high requirements. 30 is the minimum requirement, some students here have done more than 50). Students feel very confident after they graduate. The program is also very research heavy. UAB gets the National Institutes of Health (NIH) grant almost every year. The faculty is constantly doing some or the other research and will encourage students to perform research and also practice evidence-based dentistry."
Preference for citizen/GC (green card) holders	YES

Ability to take Boards at school's location?	YES
Notable alumni or faculty?	"Here you can learn from dentists like Dr. Nate Lawson, Dr. Anthony Morlandt and Dr. Basma who are all full-time faculty at the school."
Requirements	INBDE, ADAT (accepted), ECE, TOEFL
Website	https://www.uab.edu/dentistry/home/academics/idp

2. Herman Ostrow School of Dentistry at University of Southern California

Class size	34
Cost of living	Average cost of a 1 bed 1 bathroom (1b1b) apartment: $1545/-
Length of program	24 months
Preference for citizen/GC holders	NO
Requirements	INBDE, ADAT (accepted), ECE/WES, TOEFL
Website	https://dentistry.usc.edu/educational-programs/advanced-standing-program-for-international-dentists-dds/

3. University of California San Francisco School of Dentistry

Integration	"In the first year, you are fully integrated with traditional DDS candidates. In the second year, IDP (International Dental Program) students work sep-arately at Buchanan and get assistants to work with. They are quite independent in that regard. A couple of times every week, they go to the main campus at Parnassus for didactics."
Class size	20

City life and cost of living	"San Francisco is one of the most beautiful cities in the world. However, it is expensive to live in. The surrounding areas are expensive too; however, pockets can always be found in and around the city that are compatible with student affordability. San Francisco also happens to be connected to the rest of the Bay Area by public transport. Many students live in the South or East Bay and commute to the city for dental school." Average cost of a 1 bed 1 bathroom (1b1b) apartment: $2639/-
Length of program	24 months
What is special about the program?	"It is a relaxed, no-stress environment yet one that was well structured. Great balance between classes and clinics. I had enough time to do things I've never had the time to do. And the faculty is wonderful!"
Preference for citizen/GC holders	NO
Ability to take Boards at this location?	YES
Notable faculty?	Dr. Jyoti Singh
Requirements	INBDE, ECE/WES, TOEFL
Website	https://dentistry.ucsf.edu/programs/international-dentist-pathway

4. University of California Los Angeles (UCLA) School of Dentistry

Integration	YES
Class size	25

City life and cost of living	"I think for me, one of the best parts of going to UCLA would have to be living in Westwood. I was very fortunate to go to school with some of my closest friends and we all had a blast being in LA. LA is not a cheap city to live in, and even more expensive as a student. But we all managed to make the most of our time there enjoying what the city has to offer. It didn't hurt that I was only 20 minutes from Santa Monica and so going to the beach was a de-stressor!" Average cost of a 1 bed 1 bathroom (1b1b) apartment rental: $1545/-
Length of program	25 months
What is special about the program?	"Of course, the program itself at UCLA was very strong, but I would have to say I was definitely very starstruck when I met Dr. Carranza and Dr. Richard Stevenson. Having read their books, it was surreal to meet these faculty in person and even get taught by them. Also, I loved the fact that some of our clinical faculty ran practices in Beverly Hills. I was fortunate to shadow Dr. Larry Kozek at his practice and be mentored by him during the program." —Dr. Kanika Sabhlok, 2017 graduate of UCLA PPID (Professional Program for International Dentists)
Preference for citizen/GC holders	NO
Ability to take Boards at this location?	YES
Requirements	Parts I and II/INBDE and ECE, TOEFL
Website	https://www.dentistry.ucla.edu/learning/professional-program-international-dentists

5. Loma Linda University School of Dentistry (LLUSD)

Integration	"IDP (International Dentist Program) and traditional batches were partially integrated till 2021. Most of the lectures for Occlusion, Prosthodontics, Implantology, and Periodontics delivered to IDP students were of more advanced/graduate level. This is because our IDP Director treats them as practicing dentists from their respective countries and is very protective of them. The clinical floor and clinical faculty were common for IDP and traditional students."
Class size	32
Length of program	27 months
City life and cost of living	"The campus is very student friendly, and the people are extremely generous and kind. There are many affordable rental options both on campus and off campus. Furnishing the rental is free, thanks to the volunteer based *white house* from which you can get whatever you need to furnish your place, big or small. There are many vegetarian dining options on campus too where you can get delicious burritos for a dollar. Student organizations host multiple events every month, and that covers many meals. If you are looking for fancy multicuisine restau-rants, nightclubs, farmers markets, or organic avocado ice creams then downtown Redlands is the place to be; that is 5 miles from the campus. The university has a huge recreation and wellness center named Drayson center that promotes physical, emotional, and spiritual wholeness. Cost of living can range from $600-1500/-per month depending on the location of the rental and single versus family occupancy.

	During the 24-hour sabbath that the city observes, people take a break from any work-related activity. If you enjoy the outdoors then you will find many hiking trails around the campus. Not to forget that places like Palm Springs, beach cities like Huntington, Laguna, Newport beach, San Diego, and LA are just 60-75 mins drive away from the campus!"
What is special about the program?	"Students at LLUSD get a lot of exposure to Advanced Prosthodontics and Implantology cases including the opportunity to place and restore multiple implants. I restored 8-10 implants at LLUSD and placed 30-32 crowns. We also do quite a lot of digital dentistry including digital dentures, cerec, and 3shape Trios crowns!"
Preference for citizen/GC holders	"Until 2021, there was no preference for GC (green card) holders/residents. The school has many helpful resources on immigration, lodging, health insurance, etc. when it comes to taking care of students on a visa."
Ability to take Boards at this location?	YES
Notable alumni or faculty?	"Dr. Mahmoud Torabinejad (of Endo MTA fame), Dr. Jaime Lozada (past president of American Board of Implant Dentistry), Dr. Joseph Kan (implantology), Dr. Charles Goodacre (Prosthodontics), Dr. Richard Young (Injection moulding), Dr. P Young (Kois), Dr. Bakland (Trauma and Endodontics/ author of Ingles Endodontics), and Dr. L Arnett (Periodontal classification)"
Requirements	INBDE, ADAT, ECE/WES, TOEFL
Website	https://home.llu.edu/programs/dentistryinternational-dentist-program-dds

6. University of the Pacific Arthur A. Dugoni School of Dentistry

Integration	NO
Class size	26
City life and cost of living	"When I was at school between 2015-2017, there was a wide variety of housing available. If you want to live 5 mins away from school, you could be spending about $4000+ for a 1BR apartment. However, with BART (Bay Area Rapid Transit) you can live further away. I lived close to the Daly City BART station and paid about $2700/-. I also knew someone who lived as far as the Fremont/Walnut Creek area. BART makes it very convenient to live further away."
Length of program	24 months
What is special about the program?	"Humanistic model of education: emphasizing lesser student-to-doctor ratio, where students are referred to as doctors from day one, and teachers are considered mentors rather than instructors."
Preference for citizen/GC holders	NO
Ability to take Boards at this location?	"WREB (Western Regional Examining Board) is offered at school. And we also have licensing without boards available in California."
Notable alumni?	"Dr. Tiller, Gonzales, Sadowsky, Curtis, too many for me to name, not only faculty but also we had great support staff. For example, my group coordinator, Gigi. She made life so easy for us. Insurance billing and front desk schedulers were important too." —2017 graduate of IDS (International Dental Studies).
Requirements	NBDE parts I and II/INBDE, ECE, TOEFL
Website	https://dental.pacific.edu/dental/academic-programs/international-dental-studies

Disclaimer: the author is Faculty at the University of Pacific, Arthur A. Dugoni School of Dentistry at the time of this writing.

7. Western University of Health Sciences College of Dental Medicine

Integration	"Our international cohort starts with an 11-week boot camp and then integrates with the rest of the class D3 (third year of dental school) onward."
Class size	5
City life and cost of living	"Living in Pomona is very cheap compared to neighboring cities." Average cost of 1b1b rental: $1210/-
Length of program	26 months
What is special about the program?	"The most important thing is that there is no specialty program, so we get to do all the cases. We do not refer unless it is very complicated and takes a considerable amount of time (more than the two-year program time limit)." —Dr. Andy Tawfik, 2022 candidate
Preference for citizen/GC holders	YES
Ability to take Boards?	YES
Notable alumni or faculty?	"Dr. Alejandro Urdaneta (Prosthodontist), Dr. Shahrazad Aarup (IDP Course Director), and Dr. David Carlisle (IDP Managing Partner)"
Requirements	NBDE parts I and II/INBDE, WES, ADAT (accepted), TOEFL
Website	https://prospective.westernu.edu/dentistry/dmd-idp/

8. University of Colorado School of Dental Medicine

Integration	NO
Class size	40
City life and cost of living	"It is beautiful out there. You can wake up and fall asleep with a view of the mountains all the time. Most students live on campus; others live closer to Downtown Denver (15 mins away) or other suburbs and get to school by car. If you stay on campus, the cost of living is high, around $1,000 per month. You can work on campus part time to support yourself. The closest grocery store to campus is a 7-Eleven. You could get Instacart delivered, too, though."
Length of program	24 months
What is special about the program?	1. "You graduate from the program in January. This can be an advantage because you are entering the job market at a time when there aren't as many others looking for jobs." 2. "Approachability of faculty" 3. "Selection process remains fair. They don't care how many candidates are from a single country; they pick you if you're good." 4. "It's an affordable school to go to."
Preference for citizen/GC holders	NO
Ability to take Boards?	NO. One needs to fly out to another city to sit the exam.
Requirements	INBDE or NBDE parts I and II, ECE, TOEFL
Website	https://dental.cuanschutz.edu/ prospective-students/programs-of-study/ advanced-standing-international-student-program

9. Howard University (HU) College of Dentistry

Class size	Up to 10
City life and cost of living	"Washington, DC, was very nice to live in. Cost of living was acceptable." Average cost of 1b1b rental: $1469/-
Length of program	24 months
What is special about the program?	"HU Dental School is situated in a low-income part of the city. As a result, we were exposed to a variety of treatments in all aspects of dentistry. "We had professors who went beyond their line of duties to support us."
Preference for citizen/GC holders	NO
Ability to take Boards?	YES
Requirements	INBDE or NBDE part I and II, ECE or WES, TOEFL
Website	http://healthsciences.howard.edu/education/colleges/dentistry/programs/predoctoral-programs/international-dentist-program

10. Nova Southeastern University College of Dental Medicine

This is a brand-new program for foreign trained dentists at the time of this writing. For more information, contact the school directly.

11. University of Florida College of Dentistry

Class size	Up to 2
Length of program	Four years. One would start and graduate from the program with traditional DDS applicants.
Preference for citizen/GC holders	Only US citizens or green card holders can apply; Florida state residents are preferred.
Requirements	DAT, TOEFL, ADAT, ECE or WES
Website	https://admissions.dental.ufl.edu/iedp/programs-application-process/4-year-d-m-d-program/

12. University of Illinois at Chicago College of Dentistry

Integration	"Integrated from the second semester onwards; the first is all preclinical and focused on Advanced Standing students only."
Class size	Up to 52
City life, Cost of living	"Living in the city is expensive, so if you can share, it'll make things affordable. A lot of my classmates also commuted from the suburbs. Student safety is well managed due to campus police and multiple apps." Average cost of 1b1b rental: $1137/-
Length of program	28 months
What is special about the program?	"Faculty work hard to create a very friendly environment for students."
Preference for citizen/GC holders	YES
Ability to take Boards?	YES
Notable faculty	"Dr. Semprum"

Requirements	ECE, INBDE or parts I and II, TOEFL
Website	https://dentistry.uic.edu/programs/doctor-of-dental-medicine-advanced-standing-dmd-as/

13. Southern Illinois University School of Dental Medicine

Class size	Minimum 6
Length of program	Minimum 27 months
Requirements	ADAT (accepted), ECE, INBDE or parts I and II, TOEFL
Website	https://www.siue.edu/dental/iapp/

14. Indiana University School of Dentistry

Class size	14
Length of program	Minimum of 30 months
Preference for citizen/GC holders	Only US citizens, GC holders, and valid visa holders are accepted into this program.
Requirements	INBDE or parts I and II, ECE, TOEFL
Website	https://dentistry.iu.edu/admissions/how-to-apply/international-dentist-program.html

15. University of Iowa College of Dentistry and Dental Clinics

Class size	Up to 4
Length of program	30 months
Requirements	INBDE or parts I and II, ECE, TOEFL
Website	https://www.dentistry.uiowa.edu/advanced-standing-program

16. University of Maryland School of Dentistry

Class size	Dependent on space availability
Requirements	Does not participate in CAAPID so apply directly to the school. ECE or WES, TOEFL, NBDE parts I and II or INBDE
Website	https://www.dental.umaryland.edu/admissions/programs/doctor-of-dental-surgery/admission-with-advanced-standing/admission-with-advanced-standing-international-students/

17. Boston University (BU) Henry M. Goldman School of Dental Medicine

Integration	"We have almost all classes with D2 or D3 except for a few that are only for Advanced Standing (AS). For example, we have a treatment planning class with operative faculty, which is only for AS."
Class size	85
City life and cost of living	"There is a big focus on digital dentistry in BU. We have CEREC at every alternate bay. The same goes for microscopes in pre-clinics, which we learned how to use from the beginning of the course. BU has an amazing communication workshop, facial injectables for students, and a unique implant bundle, which is very cost-effective for patients. In this bundle, a patient can get an implant placed and restored for $1,000/- (total)." —2022 AS candidate Average cost of 1b1b rental: $1836/-
Length of program	24 months

What is special about the program?	"Boston is a very beautiful city with brownstone buildings, Charles River by the side if you want to relax and unwind, excellent transportation system (a rare find in the US), a lot of young people since we have so many universities within a mile's radius. Cost of living is high, but it is manageable by either sharing an apartment with classmates or BU off-campus housing."
Preference for citizen/GC holders	NO
Ability to take Boards?	YES "We have faculty who are on the exam committee. (I forgot for how many years; my guess is over ten). We give boards at BU, and since ADEX (American Board of Dental Examiners) is all manikin-based now, there is no need for live patients as of this year. We also have slots saved for the WREB (Western Regional Examination Board) or Canadian dental board exam depending on the number of candidates who want to take those exams."
Notable alumni or faculty?	"There are so many amazing faculty members in BU that I can't name them all here. Top on the list is Dr. McManama and Dr. Ferriero."
Requirements	INBDE or parts I and II, ECE, ADAT (accepted), TOEFL
Website	https://www.bu.edu/dental/admissions/as/

18. Tufts University School of Dental Medicine

Integration	YES
Class size	25–35
City life and cost of living	"Boston is the educational capital of the world. We have it all—culture, architecture, snow—and it is always a great time to go sailing!" Average cost of 1b1b rental: $1836/-
Length of program	29 months

What is special about the program?	"Diversity and having a program director specifically for the IS (International Student) class has been great. Professors want you to succeed and will always uplift you. It's a place for growth and development."
Preference for citizen/GC holders	YES
Requirements	ECE or WES, INBDE or parts I and II, TOEFL
Website	https://dental.tufts.edu/academics/dental -international-student-program

19. University of Michigan (U of M) School of Dentistry

Integration	YES
Class size	20
City life and cost of living	"Ann Arbor is like any other college town. Very vibrant, lively, and has an intellectual vibe that adds to its charm. It is one of the more expensive places to live in Michigan, but frankly, it's way cheaper compared to bigger cities like Boston or San Francisco." Average cost of 1b1b rental: $1063/-
Length of program	28 months
What is special about the program?	"U of M has been rated as the number one program for dentistry in the United States, and it happens to be one of the cheapest programs for foreign-trained dentists. One of the best things about this program that stood out to me was that in the final year, all students get three months of community dental clinic experience, which gives them a taste of real-world dentistry."
Preference for citizen/GC holders	NO

Ability to take Boards?	"At U of M, one could take CDCA (Commission on Dental Competency Assessments) boards but not WREB. However, the school supports the students taking WREB every step of the way by providing assistants, equipment, and instruments needed for the exam." —2019 graduate of U of M
Requirements	ADAT, INBDE or parts I and II, ECE, TOEFL
Website	https://www.dent.umich.edu/education/ internationally-trained-dentist-program-itdp

20. University of Minnesota (UMN) School of Dentistry

Integration	"Not integrated in the first semester, but after that, yes."
Class size	20
Length of program	29 months
What is special about the program?	1. Only school in the US where you can also sit for the Canadian licensing exam. 2. 10-week outreach program where students get to work with an assistant and practice in rural areas as well as in the Twin Cities.

	"The school projected the cost of living at \$15,000 per year, which was pretty accurate for a single person like me. My rent in a 2 bed 1 bath apartment I shared with a close friend was \$500/month at the time. This was seven years ago, so please check the latest projected costs. Bottom line, the cost of living was very reasonable, which is the case with most Midwestern cities compared to cities on either coast. The city was quite affordable. Initially, though, I was converting every US dollar into INR (Indian Rupee), and everything seemed expensive. It took me a few months before I could comfortably buy a cup of coffee at Caribou Coffee (a local Minnesotan chain of cafes), but that was a personal hang-up that I think most people have when they first move. I lived a very simple life and was aware of my finances. Being frugal helps, even for a few years after graduation.
City life and cost of living	"I felt very safe in Minneapolis. I lived close to the campus and could bike or take the bus to get to cam-pus. The campus had a walking buddy system if you wanted someone to walk you home if you were at the university after hours to study or to work in the lab.
	"Minnesotans are very outdoorsy folks and probably the healthiest Midwesterners in the country. They are also very polite and sometimes hard to read. I did make friends with regular DDS students since our class of international dentists was integrated with them within a few months of starting the program. My favorite experiences were biking the beautiful trails, attending the beer fest every year, exploring the many lakes, and attending Indian parties during the festival season. Summers are greatly cherished as Minnesota has one of the harshest winters in the country. This is something you can brag about once you have lived to tell the tale."

Preference for citizen/GC holders	"UMN does not have a restriction as to who can apply to their advanced standing program. I was on a student visa (F1) and did not have issues with immigration. In our batch of 11 international dentists, three of us were on F1 visas."
Ability to take Boards?	YES
Notable alumni?	"The program director for the PASS program (Program for Advanced Standing Students) used to be Dr. Berthold. He had started and successfully ran the same program at UPenn (University of Pennsylvania) for over 20 years before moving to the University of Minnesota to do the same. He had an intimate knowledge of dental education across the world. When he interviewed me, he knew the strengths and weaknesses of my dental school in India. I was impressed with his depth of knowledge and glad that I had not embellished my SOP (Statement of Purpose)/CV (Curriculum vitae). He was a great resource for us, and even though he has since retired, he set the grounds for a successful program that the university runs to this day." —2014 graduate of UMN, Dr. Smita Kumar, IG @ dr.smitakumar
Requirements	INBDE or parts I and II, ECE, TOEFL
Website	https://www.dentistry.umn.edu/degrees-programs/umn-pass

21. Creighton University School of Dentistry

Class size	This is a space-available program, which means that there must be an available spot in the sophomore class.
Length of program	It is a three-year program that starts in the sophomore year (in May).

What is special about the program?	"Emphasis on teaching CAD-CAM technology."
Preference for citizen/GC holders	NO
Ability to take Boards?	YES. You can sit the CDCA and WREB at the school.
Requirements	NBDE part I/INBDE, TOEFL, completion of a master's program in a dental discipline in the US
Website	https://dentistry.creighton.edu/future-students/how-apply/advanced-standing-program

22. University of Nebraska Medical Center College of Dentistry

Class size	4–6
Length of program	29 months
Requirements	INBDE or parts I and II, ECE or WES, TOEFL
Website	https://www.unmc.edu/dentistry/programs/advanced-standing/index.html

23. University of Nevada, Las Vegas School of Dental Medicine

Class size	Up to 8
Length of program	24 months
Requirements	ADAT, ECE, INBDE or NBDE parts I and II, TOEFL
Website	https://www.unlv.edu/degree/dds

24. University of New England College of Dental Medicine

Class size	1—based on space availability
Length of program	29 months
Requirements	ADAT, INBDE or parts I and II, TOEFL, ECE or WES

Website	https://www.une.edu/dentalmedicine/program/ advanced-standing-track-foreign-trained-dentists

25. Rutgers School of Dental Medicine

Integration	YES
Class size	35
Length of program	27 months
Ability to take Boards?	YES
Requirements	ADAT, INBDE or parts I and II, ECE or WES, TOEFL
Website	https://sdm.rutgers.edu/admissions/application-international-dentist-procedure.htm

26. Columbia University College of Dental Medicine, New York, NY

Class size	15
Length of program	30 months
Requirements	NBDE parts I and II/INBDE, TOEFL, ECE or WES
Website	https://www.dental.columbia.edu/education/ advanced-standing-program-foreign-trained-dentists

27. New York University College of Dentistry

Class size	20-30
City life and cost of living	"Cost of sharing a room with another person near school is around $1,500, and the cost of living is not less than $500 per month."
Length of program	28 months
What is special about the program?	"NYU was very diverse; living in NYC was great. You have the opportunity to make great connections."

Preference for citizen/GC holders	"With a similar resume, of course preference is with someone with GC, but other factors in the resume are important too." —2020 Advanced Standing graduate
Requirements	INBDE or NBDE parts I and II, TOEFL, ECE
Website	https://dental.nyu.edu/academicprograms/dds-program/advanced-standing.html

28. University at Buffalo (UB) School of Dental Medicine

Integration	"Program at UB is fully integrated with traditional DDS students. There's a summer program from the end of May to the start of August where IDP (International Dental Program) students are on their own, and they are prepared for the integration with the 3rd year students. During the summer program, we must pass several skill tests. After that all classes are held with traditional students. There were 116 students in my class, 26 IDPs and 90 traditional students."
Class size	24
City life and cost of living	"Buffalo is a beautiful, small city, with lots of scenic places to visit, and very close to Canada and NYC of course. There's some crime reports from time to time, but security is good. Cost of living is very doable. The 1 BHK I rented was for $1100/-. It came with good maintenance service."
Length of program	24 months
What is special about the program?	"You get a good mix of patients since it is the only school in the city. Faculty members and staff in administration are super nice and helpful. They help students at every step whether it is career related or personal. Faculty is world renowned."
Preference for citizen/GC holders	"During my time, I did not see a preference for GC/citizenship, everyone was given an equal chance."

Notable alumni or faculty?	"Special shout out to Dr. Gambacorta and Dr. Shenoy, they really care about the students and are pillars of the school, without them I can't imagine the IDP program being a huge success." —2018 IDP graduate
Requirements	INBDE or parts I and II, ECE, TOEFL
Website	http://dental.buffalo.edu/education/dds-program/dds-program/international-dentist-program.html

29. University of North Carolina, Chapel Hill, Adam's School of Dentistry

Class size	8
Length of program	29 months
Requirements	INBDE or parts I and II, ECE, TOEFL
Website	https://dentistry.unc.edu/aspid/

30. University of Oklahoma College of Dentistry

Class size	14
Length of program	29 months
Requirements	ECE and INBDE or parts I and II, TOEFL
Website	https://dentistry.ouhsc.edu/Academic-Programs/Advanced-Standing-for-International-Dentists-ASPID

31. University of Pennsylvania School of Dental Medicine

Class size	35–40
Length of program	29 months
Preference for citizen/GC holders	NO
Requirements	INBDE or parts I and II, ECE, TOEFL
Website	https://www.dental.upenn.edu/admissions-academics/program-for-advanced-standing-students/

32. University of Pittsburgh ('Pitt') School of Dental Medicine

Integration	"The classes for international students at the University of Pittsburgh were completely integrated with the regular classes. However, there is a summer semester we have to pass before admission is guaranteed."
Class size	Up to 8
City life and cost of living	"Pittsburgh is a medium-sized city where sports is a religion. They have a very diverse food scene, the museums are plenty and beautiful, and with your student pass, you have the luxury of free admission to any of the museums and botanical gardens. You also get a free bus pass so one can explore the city, including the parks and casinos. The cost of living is average; one can find a shared room near the campus for less than $1,000/-, and there are other options as well."
Length of program	24 months
What is special about the program?	"Since the dental school shares the building with a pharmacy school and it is right across from the hospitals, the inter-professional interaction and the opportunity to learn from each other is ample. Pitt is proud of its special-needs department, which provides dental services to people with special needs under general anesthesia in-house. They also have an esteemed anesthesia program and give you the opportunity to be certified in IV sedation while you are a dental student."
Preference for citizen/GC holders	NO
Ability to take Boards?	YES

Notable alumni or faculty?	"The International Dentist Program (IDP) would not be possible without Dr. Potluri, who is the head of the radiology department and the director of the IDP program. She is available for guidance, support, and mentorship throughout the program." —2018 advanced standing graduate
Requirements	ADAT, ECE, INBDE or parts I and II, TOEFL
Website	https://www.dental.pitt.edu/education/international-advanced-standing-program

33. Temple University Kornberg School of Dentistry

Class size	They offer two programs. Two-year program: 10 seats Three-year program: based on availability
Length of program	Two years or three years
Requirements	ADAT, ECE, INBDE or parts I and II, TOEFL
Website	https://www.temple.edu/academics/degree-programs/international-dentists-dmd-dn-dnft-dmd

34. University of Puerto Rico, School of Dental Medicine

Class size	10
Length of program	25 months
What is special about the program?	"This program is open to US citizens, permanent residents, as well as international students but is mainly targeted to dentists with dental degrees from Spanish-speaking international dental schools. Proficiency in the Spanish language will be assessed during the interview process."
Requirements	Must be proficient in the Spanish language, TOEFL, INBDE or parts I and II, ECE
Website	https://dental.rcm.upr.edu/advanced-placement-program/

35. Meharry Medical College School of Dentistry

Class size	10
Length of program	24 months
Requirements	ADAT, TOEFL, INBDE or parts I and II, ECE or WES
Website	https://home.mmc.edu/school-of-dentistry/

36. University of Texas Health Science Center at Houston School of Dentistry

Integration	YES
Class size	Advanced Standing applicants will be considered for admission only if space is available in the second-year DDS class. This school does not participate in CAAPID.
Length of program	Three years
What is special about the program?	"Applicants must not have been out of the predoctoral dental school for more than five years at the time of acceptance or must have completed a two-year post-doctoral program accredited by the ADA within the past five years or have successfully completed a pre-ceptorship program at UTHealth School of Dentistry within the past five years."
Requirements	NBDE part I/INBDE, TOEFL
Website	https://dentistry.uth.edu/students/doctor-of-dental-surgery/index.htm

37. University of Texas Health Science Center at San Antonio School of Dentistry

Class size	8–10. This program does not participate in CAAPID.
Requirements	INBDE or parts I and II, ECE, TOEFL
Website	https://www.uthscsa.edu/academics/dental/programs/international-dentist-program

38. Virginia Commonwealth University School of Dentistry

Class size	10
Length of program	33 months
Requirements	ADAT, INBDE or parts I and II, ECE, or WES
Website	https://dentistry.vcu.edu/programs/ internationaldentists/

39. University of Washington (UW) School of Dentistry

Integration	YES
Class size	10
City life and cost of living	"Seattle is a city for everyone. Booklovers, outdoor enthusiasts, and seafood connoisseurs can easily find a community here. I liked the area so much I continued to practice in the city after graduation. Affordable student housing is easy to find if you look on Craigslist and ask around in your network. I got super lucky and found a 2BHK with my friend near the bus line to school for $1200/- per month. We lived there for 2 years and loved it!"
Length of program	27
What is special about the program?	"Our DECOD (Dental Education in the Care for People with Disabilities) center offers a one-of-a-kind teaching program at the school. All dental students learn how to better support and treat children and adults with special needs in a dental setting while also managing their medical considerations. "Seattle is well known for dental continuing education; UW has ties with all the major Study Clubs in the area, including the Tucker Gold Study Club and Academy of General Dentistry that host a variety of world-renowned lecturers in the city. Students get access to many of these programs for free or at a reduced cost. I took the Cast Gold elective twice with Dr. Tucker Jr. in my final year. The lessons learned during that time were invaluable for my career."

Preference for citizen/GC holders	NO
Ability to take Boards at this location?	YES
Notable alumni and faculty?	''Drs. Chan and Paranjpe are the pillars of our IDDS community!''
Requirements	INBDE or parts I and II, ECE, TOEFL
Website	https://dental.washington.edu/students/dds-programs/international-dds-program/

Disclaimer: Author is a 2018 graduate of the UW IDDS program.

40. Marquette University School of Dentistry

Class size	Dependent on space availability
Length of program	36 months
Requirements	ADAT, INBDE or parts I and II, TOEFL, ECE
Website	https://www.marquette.edu/dentistry/admissions/international-students.php

TIPS TO REMEMBER FOR EVERY SCHOOL

Selection Process

Here is some advice from Daniel Chan, DDS, a faculty member at the University of Washington and past director of the IDDS (International DDS) program. He says the following regarding the selection process that UW employs for its candidates:

We have two layers of selection. First, the committee looks at all the paper documentation. They check if scores, letters of recommendation, statement of purpose, etc., are all complete and present. Statement of purpose is the number one thing we are looking at. We don't want something standardized or copied. We are looking for your personal goals and your vision. We weigh on the statement of purpose quite heavily.

Second is the review conducted by faculty who you meet in person when you are selected for an interview. They look for communication and leadership skills in you. What kind of doctor, colleague, and teacher will you be in the future? They look at the way you talk and present yourself.

Do schools ever see red flags in candidates?

According to Dr. Chan:

Yes. Indifference, lack of focus, and ethical concerns are the main red flags. There are some candidates who, based on their statement of purpose and their interview, appear as though they have a right to be accepted, most likely because they are getting funded by their government. They think this matters to us, and we will accept them because of that. This couldn't be further from the truth. In the US, everyone is treated the same. Getting a scholarship doesn't matter. We only look at the candidate's overall competency.

How do faculty know they chose the right candidate?

Dr. Chan says:

We have always had 100% of you passing the clinical boards at UW. This is a source of major pride for us. Several of you shine in community service outside the school, and we see you giving back in various ways. Many of you understand the importance of education and volunteer as faculty at the school, and that makes us very happy. All of you are not only interested in getting but also in giving back. This highlights character and helps us feel we chose the right candidates.

Letters of Recommendation (LOR)

It is a common understanding amongst most foreign-trained dentists that at least one letter of recommendation, from a total of three, needs to be from a school professor (apart from the Dean). Dr. Chan responds:

That is not true. We are looking for a letter from someone who can vouch for your character and clinical skills closer to the time you apply. Do we want a letter from a professor who taught you fifteen years ago? No.

Many students who have left their home country many years ago may find it difficult to get a LOR from their professors or their Dean. If all they can get is a letter without passionate support for the candidate, then seeking in-depth letters from local professionals may be a better choice.

If there is a dentist around town, close to the university you are applying to, who has observed how you work as a den-tal assistant or as their mentee, etc., that will be huge for us because there is nothing quite like it. This is because it means that your character and clinical skills have already been vouched for by someone we know.

If you have a letter from a prominent dentist in another country, but nobody knows them here, it wouldn't matter as much. The person who writes the letter, in this case, is gener-ally less important than the content of the letter.

Every letter gets a score. Some of us work as arbitrators or tiebreakers in this process. Please remember this is tedious and time-consuming for us as well.

Statement of Purpose (SOP)
Dhara Patel, D3, at UW, reminds candidates:

Focus on making your SOP unique and illustrate who you are as a person. Some schools don't have a supplemental applica-tion, so the SOP is all they get to read about you. In my first cycle, I wrote about everything I did as an MPH student in my SOP. In my second cycle, I realized that schools could read my CV to know what I did during my MPH. I should instead tell them what I can bring to the school as a DDS candidate. Don't brag about things you have done in the past; show them what you could bring to the school in the future.

4

GAP YEAR: BETWEEN DENTAL SCHOOL ABROAD AND DENTAL SCHOOL IN THE US

"I finished dental school many years ago. Now, what?"

You finished dental school a while ago, are out in the workforce, or already in America and looking for ways to improve your candidacy. What can you do now to add to your experience and knowledge base?

COMMUNITY SERVICE

One of the most meaningful things we can do with our time is to give it back to the community. As healthcare providers, we have recognized that natural call and made it our profession. Many of us volunteer at community clinics, homeless shelters, and elderly homes on a weekly basis. Continue doing the same while waiting for an interview. If you initiated a special project while volun-teering, mention it on your statement of purpose. If you know a leader within the organization, who understands your work and can write well, ask them for a letter of recommendation.

Heads of nonprofits often understand the role of healthcare providers more intimately than anyone else. Hence, they may be more willing to help you.

ORGANIZED DENTISTRY

Join the American Dental Association. Read online blogs and resources published in ASDA (American Student Dental Association) *Contour* and *New Dentist Now,* both managed under the umbrella of the American Dental Association. Both feature articles from dental students and new dentists practicing in the US and can give you a great visual of life for you in a few years. This is a good way to get into the mindset of becoming a dental student. Many authors can also be contacted for more information, and several are willing to mentor you.

Disclaimer: Author regularly contributes to blogs in *New Dentist Now* and wrote a monthly post on the 'business side of dentistry' in 2021.

SHADOWING

A great way to learn the ins-and-outs of a dental clinic is to spend time shadowing or assisting at one. Approach all the offices in your neighborhood, including the local dental school, to try to get this experience. Mix it up and shadow at different kinds of clinics—some specialty and some general. This will help you understand what procedures you are interested in and guide you clinically. It will also help you meet with potential mentors who might help critique your bench-test prep work.

Ketan Jumani, DDS, MPH, MSD, a practicing pediatric den-tist based in Sammamish, Washington, says, "Once you come to the US, finding a place to practice for the bench test is difficult. On the weekends and after regular school hours, I would shadow dentists at various clinics to get a better understanding of how dentistry was practiced in the US. I even had some of these den-tists critique my preps and give me pointers for my bench test."

TIP: Print your resume and a small bio explaining who you are. For example: *Foreign-trained dentist looking to shadow local dentists, currently in the dental school application stage.* Call the office and say "Hi, I'm a dentist from India looking to meet your doctor. When do they take lunch? I'd love to swing by and introduce myself. I'm a prospective dental student and new to the area."

PRO TIP: If you make it past the front desk and get an appointment with the dentist, go and say, "Hey, I'd love to shadow you for a few days if that's okay or take you out for lunch and hear about your experience as a dentist in this neighborhood." Bringing macaroons for the team is always a hit. Most people are happy to honor that kind of request. Be genuine when building a relationship like this from scratch. You might be in touch with this doctor for years to come. They might even offer you a job once you become a dentist.

The doctor I shadowed when I was still giving my NBDE Part 1 ultimately became the dentist for my aunt's family. She and I are still in touch!

Many offices might need you to sign a HIPAA (Health Insurance Portability and Accountability Act) and confidentiality form. And lots of offices will say no to shadowing straight away. Don't be too disappointed when that happens. Remember, it isn't easy to let a stranger into your office and have them interact with your staff and patients. Keep trying.

READING

A lot of interviewers asked me which books I was reading. I don't think quoting academic books would have been impressive to any of them. Dentists are known to be well-rounded professionals with an enviable work-life balance. Dental school is hectic, and the faculty wants to know if you have the capacity to excel in academics and take care of your mental health and personal life, all at the same time.

They are looking into your future when they ask you what books you are reading or what hobbies you have. While working on your application is important, so is taking a break, spending time outdoors, traveling, reading, and experiencing life outside of dentistry. Give yourself that time and enjoy this journey. For tips on self-care during the stressful interview stage, head to the end of Chapter 6.

For book recommendations, check out my personal website: https://www.sampadadeshpandedds.com

ACADEMIA

Do you live close to a dental school? Consider approaching senior faculty in the school and ask them if they need help with any papers they are working on. Spend a few weeks researching specific topics you are interested in and pitch those to faculty at the school. Additionally, recruit one or two of your friends in such projects. It boosts morale and makes working towards the publishing process more fun.

GRATITUDE

This is not mentioned enough, but it is an important part of the process, and of life. Sending a thank -you card to every single person who has helped you along the way and staying in touch with them over the years via postcards or letters is important. As students, we often forget how little time faculty and practicing dentists have on their hands. *They* are doing you a favor when writing a letter of recommendation. You can easily get a stack of preprinted thank -you cards from the corner craft store and begin writing notes in them every week. This is also a way to relieve anxiety and count your blessings. So, this is not only good for the receivers of your card, but it is also good for you.

MPH

A lot of students get involved in academic programs while in their gap years. Being a student at an academic program like MPH (Master of Public Health) or MHA (Master in Health Administration) is looked at very favorably by a majority of dental school admission committees as it shows commitment, perseverance, and an interest in pursuing higher education in the United States.

Nayanika Sanga, DDS, MPH, says the following about her MPH experience at the University of Alabama at Birmingham:

> The MPH program is a wonderful way to understand the healthcare and educational system in the US and build a net-work of supporters. An MPH is essentially a public health degree that attracts a wide, diverse diaspora of profession-als—engineers, dentists, and doctors, to name a few.

> I used my MPH program to connect the dots between public health in the US and my training in clinical dentistry from India. My goal was to get admitted to a DDS program, and because I made that clear to my program mentor, she helped me connect with faculty at the dental school at UAB. These connections helped me train for my bench test and find men-tors who would later write my letters of recommenda-tion. I also firmly believe that having an MPH background makes us more informed clinicians and helps us understand clinical guidelines better.

Next is Ketan Jumani, DDS, MSD, MPH, on the reasons why he enjoyed his MPH program at John Hopkins:

> During dental school in India, I was interested in commu-nity dental health. I enjoyed conducting oral hygiene educa-tion at homeless shelters and prisons. I was also very inter-ested in tobacco cessation and filmed a few documentaries that were later used for World No Tobacco Day education.

Public health was and remains one of my passions. I was unsure about what I wanted to do after graduation in India and wasn't entirely certain about going into clinical dentistry right away. There-fore, I considered doing an MPH.

After my MPH program, I became an associate faculty mem-ber at the school, helping conduct clinical trials in infec-tious diseases, which was my concentration back then. I also supported myself by taking a job at the School of Medicine doing data entry. This experience ultimately helped me get a great LOR (Letter of Recommendation) for a DDS program.

Due to my research-heavy MPH, I had lots of poster pre-sentations. My thesis presentation was published in *JAMA* (Journal of the American Medical Association) with me as its first author. This strengthened my application for a DDS pro-gram. I got lots of questions from the interviewers about it.

CE COURSES

While you may be on a budget, remember to account a little for CE (Continuing Education) courses or poster and paper presen-tations. Use those opportunities to network with dental students, meet new dentists, find other foreign- trained colleagues, and get face time with faculty from different schools.

Get in the habit of collecting business cards and handing out your own. Stay in touch with the people you meet over email or LinkedIn. Use every email, phone conversation, or in-person meeting to have a question answered. It may be a question about your application, about the school the person attended, or about their work experience. As a prospective student, make a list of questions you are curious about. Asking the right questions, politely, leads you to a place of more awareness.

PRECEPTORSHIPS AND OBSERVERSHIP PROGRAMS

I attended the three-month OMFS (Oral & Maxillofacial Surgery) preceptorship program at UCSF (University of California San Francisco) and consider it to be one of the highlights of my gap year. I was watching live maxillofacial surgeries two or three times a week, meeting dental students and residents every day, and getting the opportunity to live in San Francisco for a few months. What was not to love?

In any of these programs, you get what you put in. During my preceptorship, I had my statement of purpose critiqued by mentors, received a letter of recommendation from my professor, worked on a research paper, and helped a few other professors in data collection. I only had three months to make this possible, so while time was critical, the experience did ultimately pay off because many schools I interviewed with that year asked me about my preceptorship.

Purely by luck, one of my faculty interviewers at UW used to be a student of the professor at UCSF who wrote my letter of recommendation. Upon reading my LOR (letter of recommenda-tion) at the interview, she immediately recognized my professor and asked me how he was doing. I'd like to think that this tipped the scales in my favor by a huge margin.

PRO TIP: We need to remember that the dental industry is very small and that most people know of each other. So always be respectful and talk fondly of your experiences with others.

APPLYING TO SCHOOLS

While the number of interview invites may differ from one can-didate to another, most prospective students agree on max-imizing their chances by applying to several schools.

Ketan Jumani, DDS, MSD, MPH, says:

> I applied to five to seven schools, most on the West Coast,
> a few on the East Coast. There are some programs that
> have a larger class size and are not fully integrated with the

tra-ditional DDS students. I was not very interested in those schools but applied to them as a backup.

I interviewed at San Antonio, UW (University of Washing-ton), Boston, and USC (University of Southern California). I was accepted at San Antonio and UW. I was invited to a few additional interviews but did not end up going because, by then, I'd already accepted UW's offer.

Although San Antonio had an equally strong clinical pro-gram, I finally chose UW because of the smaller class size (five students at the time), having specialty programs at the dental school, it being a research-heavy institution, and the opportunity to live in Seattle.

Nayanika Sanga, DDS, MPH, remarks on the importance of networking at interviews and applying to several schools in each cycle:

I interviewed throughout my time as an MPH student. In my first year, I applied late and interviewed at only three schools. In my final year, I interviewed at seven or more schools, got accepted at two, and wait-listed at the rest.

I met *you* (Sampada) at my UW interview during my first cycle, where you were a proctor, and asked you questions on how to improve my candidacy. You recommended I be the first to apply to every school because of the admissions being rolling.

I did not realize the value of putting in my applications early until the time I did what you said in my next cycle and auto-matically got more interviews. This also taught me to use interviews as a networking opportunity and meet more peo-ple, ask more questions.

Applying to a ton of schools requires juggling money orders, paperwork, and essays, along with everything else. The best advice I can give here is to organize well ahead of time and apply early.

Dhara Patel mentions the value of introspection after every cycle and the importance of asking for feedback after every rejection:

In my first cycle, I applied to fifteen schools. I wanted to give myself every opportunity possible. I later realized that some schools will never invite me for an interview, no matter what I do. So, in my second cycle, I applied to only six schools.

Many schools tend to invite residents of the state they are based in. Some schools say ADAT (Advanced Dental Admis-sions Test) is not compulsory but tend to invite only students who have taken the exam. Few schools rarely invite students who have multiple attempts on their NBDE (National Board Dental Examinations). Although they will not directly men-tion it, when you call and ask for feedback, they will mention that "most of the students we invite have cleared their boards in a single attempt." I took that as a sign and did not apply again. There are also a few schools that have the reputation of not providing enough patients for their students, mostly because of big class sizes and competition with other dental schools in the city. I decided not to apply to those schools either because I didn't want to invest time and money in a program like that.

I'd recommend that students, if in their second or third appli-cation cycle, call every school they applied to prior and ask for feedback. The feedback I got from schools proved to be crucial.

5

BENCH TEST PREPARATION

Every school has a different way of conducting interviews. Some have a comprehensive bench test; others do not. Some have a faculty and current student interview you; others have only a single faculty member interview you. Few conduct a skills assessment (that includes molding wax into different shapes), a written test (often used to prequalify you for an in-person interview), and a multiple mini-interview session with a focus on ethical questions.

The interview process either lasts a full day or more. I've been to a school that had three long days of interviewing. It calls for a lot of patience, persistence, and being on top of your game.

This section is about the often-dreaded bench examination. There are several ways to prepare for the bench test. One of the ways is by attending a professional course. There are various courses conducted all over the world that help prepare students for this important interview component. That said, remember that none of the courses mentioned below are endorsed by the ADA (American Dental Association) and that courses taken one year might not elicit the same response the next.

The goal in this section is to not recommend any specific course, as experiences can be very subjective and time sensitive. Every dentist and student interviewed for this book has mentioned a different way of preparing for the test. The path you take is ultimately your decision.

I took two of the better-known courses in the US between the years 2014 and 2015: Duggan Institute and Dr. Tools.

DUGGAN INSTITUTE

Duggan Institute is what I had heard the most about and what I had been recommended to take by almost every student who got accepted.

1. I took the ten-day course with Dr. Duggan and stayed close to the center for almost a month after to practice under his guidance.

2. With his keen sense of perfectionism, Dr. Duggan cri-tiqued my preps the way nobody else (even later in school) would. I truly believe that his critique helped me become better and helped me ace my bench tests after. I sometimes still hear his voice in my head while preparing a tooth for a crown.

3. The course had another positive benefit that I will forever be grateful for. I attended the course with fourteen other men and women. We became an uncommonly tight-knit group. Many of my colleagues from the course are very good friends of mine to this day and have been confi-dantes throughout this journey. I met many of them again at interviews the following year. Seeing a friendly face low-ered my anxiety level tremendously. It is important to realize that everyone who interviews with you is not your competitor. These people are working as hard as you, so help them when you can.

4. Even though I practiced for many days after the course ended at the teaching center, I bought the home setup to practice even more. It included a typodont and mount, hundreds of burs (you will see how quickly you burn

through them when working on plastic teeth), boxes of masks, gloves, and of course, a handpiece. Practice makes perfect.

5. I first took the course in April 2015, with no invite in hand. I was lucky to have taken the course early because just a few months later, I got interviews for Colorado, Buffalo, and UW. I was very confident going in for these interviews because of the course. Had I not taken it early, I would not have been as prepared. I went back to the center a second time before another set of interviews. I stayed close to the center and practiced from 9 AM to 5 PM, 6 days a week. Not only was I getting my work critiqued every day, I was also meeting prospective students who were taking the course with Dr. Duggan at the center. Many of these students are good friends now, and several were interviewed for this book. We are a very friendly and supportive community.

DR. TOOLS

1. I took this course in early 2014, right before my first interview, and with only one month of preparation time ahead. TIP: No matter which course you take, one month of preparation time is almost never enough.

2. The number one reason many smart candidates do not get an acceptance is because they start preparing late for the bench test. They find it presumptuous to invest in instru-ments, typodonts, etc. when they don't have an interview invite. This was my mistake and one of the reasons why it took me so long to get an acceptance. I'd heard this advice before and ignored it. Don't let that be you. Give yourself enough time to prepare for the bench. Schools like UW weigh heavily on the results of their bench test.

3. The course at the time involved two days of in-depth training. After the course, you retain the ability to practice at the clinic in one of several operatories and show Dr. Sandhu your work to get feedback.

PRO TIP: I found the biggest value in taking the course at Duggan Institute first, practicing at his teaching center for a month after and then practicing with Dr. Sandhu at her clinic later for revision.

KEY TAKEAWAY

Start preparing right away, and do not wait for an interview call to spur you into action. Most of our colleagues attending inter-views have been preparing for months in advance. Some have been preparing for years—no joke. Know that you're competing with smart, motivated, and extremely competent people. Do not take it lightly, or you'll be wasting an interview opportunity.

Dhara Patel shares a similar experience on the bench test:

I was invited to UW for two cycles. In the first cycle, I under-estimated the bench test, not knowing it was a very tough test. When I met other interviewees and realized how expe-rienced and prepared they were, I knew right away I was not going to ace the test and needed professional help.

After my first cycle, I signed up for Stevenson's bench test course. It was a game-changer for me. I initially wanted to take his seven-day course, but it was already full. So, I took his three-day course instead. I highly recommend it.

Practice for the bench test from the beginning; do not wait for the invite. You usually get an invite a few weeks prior to the interview. Sometimes, if you have been wait-listed, you get an invite a week before the test. Don't wait. Prac-tice every day. Most schools ask for an upper maxilla prep, so start working with indirect vision. This requires time and consis-tent practice.

For further information on bench test preparation and school applications, reach out directly to Dhara at drdhara124@ gmail.com

Nayanika Sanga, DDS, did not take a bench prep course. She says:

I decided to trust my instinct and mentors. I was on good talking terms with my prosthodontics professor in India and had him heavily critique my bench prep work over virtual meetings. I had also built a strong set of coaches during my MPH and friends who were already admitted in advanced standing programs who would critique my work and suggest ways to improve my operator position.

An important thing I'd like to share here is to not be shy. I remember asking which burs we should use for a class II cavity prep. I knew a certain set of burs from my training in India but wanted to know if those were the same ones used here in America. Be open to getting feedback from everyone.

It was early 2014 when I got my first dental school interview. I was excited about finally getting an invite. At the same time, I was concerned because I had only two months to prepare and had not yet practiced on mannequins for the bench testing component. Truth is, I couldn't have been any less prepared.

Moral of the story? Prepare early.

NOTE: As of 2020, the global pandemic led to a change to the in-person bench examination. Many schools are now conducting virtual examinations. Do not hesitate to reach out to the school with specific questions on what to expect in an interview.

6

PERSONAL INTERVIEW

Before we dive into personal interviews and how to prepare for them, here is some advice for interacting with other candidates. Yes, other candidates. A common mistake many interviewees make is not to interact with their colleagues during an interview. They think of other interviewees as competition and keep to themselves throughout this time.

If you plan on doing this, you are missing out on camaraderie, advice, and potential friendships. These are your future colleagues, people who you will meet at other interviews too. They can help you get better. Sharing resources will only strengthen our small community of foreign-trained dentists. It will not detract from your goals.

The people I met at interviews became my friends. Over the years, we have all helped each other grow and succeed. We have helped each other find associateships, answered questions on immigration, attended dental conferences together, and invited each other's families home for dinner.

A mistake I made in the beginning was spending a lot of time preparing for the bench test alone and little to none on the personal interview. Both are crucial parameters for success. Colleagues applying with you to dental school are just as quali-fied, if not more credentialed, than you. Some have years of work experience, and others have PhDs and multiple publications. Sharpen your communication skills and get ready to shine.

Body Language And Interview Preparation

Your interview is the one fighting chance you get to wow everyone you meet and build relationships with teachers, students, and future colleagues. Even if you don't get accepted at the school, these are your colleagues, and all of them deserve your love and attention. When I was in my second cycle of applications, I was nervous and kept mostly to myself. I later realized how uptight and rude I might have appeared. Body language is something we give very little credit to, but it is as important as the rest of the interview.

It is important to smile, mingle with other candidates, and ask the right questions. One thing that helped me prepare better for interviews was working with a coach to improve my delivery. For recommendations on coaches, please head to my website: https://www.sampadadeshpandedds.com and search for 'coach'. My coach taught me how to craft moving stories to enlist what I have done in the past without sounding conceited. I use this communication tool to this day while interacting with patients.

Sometimes, personal interviews can help make up for average bench test scores. Daniel Chan, DDS, says, "We are looking for people who are coachable and have excellent clinical skills. Our bench test results are extremely important to us. If you've failed in most bench test areas, it shows a lack of preparation and interest, and you will not be considered a serious candidate." He continues, "However, all that said, the bench test is a barrier. You have to get at least a minimum, pass most areas, and absolutely ace your interview."

Being Culturally And Linguistically Inclusive

Daniel Chan, DDS, shares knowledge about the criteria that they are looking for in candidates:

We have never been disappointed because of the clinical skills of our candidates. It is usually cultural differences, an inability to adjust to life in America, or when candidates are too shy to approach their classmates and patients. There was a candidate like that who was shy throughout her academic program. She found it very difficult to adjust to the culture here, and that affected her ability to become a good clinician. This was a big problem.

Most candidates who have been in the States for some time, either pursuing other academic programs or because of fam-ily immigration, etc., tend to adjust more easily to the clin-ical and academic settings here. We value gender and racial equality and champion diversity. It is important for our candi-dates to demonstrate that understanding well before applying to schools. They can generally do that by working as a dental assistant, pursuing a preceptorship or a research fellowship, etc.

Remember that a lot of these criteria can be measured in an interview. The faculty is always looking out for people who will bring value to the school as alumni.

Ketan Jumani, DDS, MSD, MPH, provides further tips to candidates preparing for interviews:

I think to be a good interviewee, you need to have confi-dence and need to be a good conversationalist. It takes years to become a good conversationalist. However, there are a few standard questions that every interviewer will ask you:

- Tell me about yourself.

- What brings you here?

- What are your strengths and interests?

- Five or ten years down the line, what are your goals?

You should expect certain questions and prepare for them. Write your responses down to these questions, practice in front of the mirror, building in some humor and pauses so that it flows naturally and does not appear very rehearsed.

Stay updated on what's happening around town and in the world. Reading a lot of books and staying updated on current events adds value to the conversation.

TYPES OF INTERVIEWS AND PREPARATION TIPS

The personal interview differs based on the school. Some schools conduct a panel interview composed of a couple of faculty only (e.g., at UW), some schools have a panel with a mix of students and faculty (e.g., University of Colorado), some have just faculty (e.g., UCSF), and others hold small sessions with only one faculty member (e.g., UCLA, Pacific).

What's common among them all? All of them are stressful and require you to be calm, collected, and confident.

TIPS that May Help You Prepare
1. Participating in mock interviews. Ask your friends or family members to interview you. Pull up frequently-asked dental school interview questions and practice getting quizzed. Ask everyone for critical feedback. Have them review your grammar, diction and frequency of "umms." Most friends would gladly help you with this.

2. Know your resume and statement of purpose well. Be prepared to share stories on leadership activities and com-munity service.

3. Use every opportunity in an interview to share something meaningful about what you can bring to the table as a future alumnus of the school.

4. Consider working with a coach, like I did.

What Most Interviews Are Trying to Determine

1. Are you a good culture fit for this program? (Are you easy to like and get along with?)

2. Are you qualified for this program? (What was your experi-ence before this? What brought you to the US? How serious are you about continuing your dental education? What are you going to do with your second round of schooling?)

3. How are you going to add to the alumni background of the school? (Why should we take you? What makes you stand out? What are your plans for the future? Are you going to practice in the area? Would you teach at the school? Would you create a different set of clinics? How would you impact your patient community?)

4. What makes you a well-rounded person? (What are your hobbies outside of dentistry? How will you pay for the program?)

5. Many schools will ask you questions that make you uncom-fortable. I was frequently asked things like, "This is your third cycle of applications. Why have you not gotten accepted anywhere yet? What is different about you this year? What have you learned about yourself during this time?" They want to see how well you take criticism and have improved your candidacy over the years.

6. Schools also want to know if you have what it takes to go through the grueling process of dental school again. They don't want candidates who will stress out about every little exam or complain about the work required or blame professors. Some of the tougher questions I got were, "Do you have any goals outside of dentistry or your career? What if you don't get to become a dentist in the US? What if no school chooses you this cycle? What are your alternate career plans?" There are no right or wrong

answers to these. They are subjective but brace yourself for questions like that. It is best to be thoroughly prepared.

Nayanika Sanga, DDS, has an additional tip for interview day:

You need to recognize your weaknesses first. The interview is going to test your physical, mental, and emotional limits. I have a ton of food allergies, and although every school did their best to accommodate my restrictions, there was always some ingredient in the food that would bring me down. And like most of us, when I'm hungry or unwell, I can't concen-trate. After recognizing this, I made sure I always carried familiar comfort food with me to interviews. (I still give credit to the tiramisu I carried for acing my Michigan bench exam.) Being well-rested and well-fed is important.

Self-Care during the Stressful Interviewing Process

Is this section important? Why did it even make it here?

Yes, this section is very important, and you will find out why very soon. Here is the deal. I wish someone had told me that it is just a matter *of time* before I got into school, and that getting stressed and anxious about it was not going to help me get there any faster.

Let me explain. I was so hyper focused on getting into dental school my first cycle of applying that when I was asked the ques-tion at one of my first interviews, "What are your goals outside of dentistry?" I blanked out for a few minutes. It was not only embarrassing that I didn't answer the question but also, I did not get accepted there. I felt saddened by the fact that I had lost my creative personality in the process of applying to dental school.

I had neglected all my hobbies, my love for reading, dancing, music, and travel, for the singular goal of getting accepted into dental school. The realization became even more apparent at the end of 2014 with 4 rejections. And I did not have any fun that year either. None of you should have to go through that because life happens only once. And while it is important for you to work towards your goals and make your dreams come true, it also means enjoying all the gifts this life has to offer to you.

While all of this may sound very philosophical, it has very real benefits and consequences. My final year of dental school applica-tions went a lot easier because I took time off to see my friends. Additionally, I traveled extensively and went on sight-seeing tours in every city I had an interview in (I didn't know when I would get to go to those cities again, so why not?), read plenty of books, and took classes in Spanish. It was an amazing year because not only did I get three acceptances that year, but I was also extremely happy and in high spirits. *That* probably showed in interviews.

So, here is a short accountability checklist for those of you preparing for interviews right now:

1. Build a group of mentors and coaches who can encourage you every time you face a rejection or are feeling demoti-vated going into an interview. For me, a lot of the time, my mentor was my mom. Hearing her uplifting tone of voice always made me feel better.

2. Take 30 mins every day to get outside for a walk, run, or bike ride. Practicing on typhodont (plastic) teeth all day indoors can be the most boring thing in the world. Make sure to get some fresh air.

3. Share your concerns and fears with a spouse or best friend. If they are not in dentistry, all the better. My non-dental friends often have the best advice when times get tough. They help me remember that there is a world outside of dentistry.

4. Consider meditating or journaling every day to exercise your mind and stay in touch with your thoughts. While I never did those things during dental school applications, I now wish I did. Those years might have gone easier. Meditation and journaling are a regular part of my day

now, and that of many, many others in dentistry. As a profession, we are burdened not just with physical and financial stressors but emotional stressors too. Meditation can be a very effective way to release pent up anxiety.

5. Eat and sleep well. A full night's rest and a happy tummy are sometimes more important than many other things.

6. Remember, that it is after all, just a matter of time before you get over this phase. *It is going to happen for you.* Believe it, manifest it. And don't give up.

7

CHOOSING A SCHOOL

Are you one of those people who got multiple acceptances? Awesome! Now, you have a big decision to make. Here's some advice on how to choose the right school.

COST

Let's face it: where you got your DDS or DMD does not matter. What matters is that you got it, and then you get licensed to finally practice and impact your community. However, the cost of an education can either cripple you or can lighten the weight on your shoulders. Consider this carefully when choosing a school. You want to be able to pay off your student loans as quickly as possible.

TIP: It becomes harder to justify a student loan upwards of $500K when you want to buy a practice and haven't yet paid off your student loan. During economic downturns, banks don't look at it kindly. Your interest rates will always be different from your friend who went to a public, lower-cost school.

PROXIMITY TO JOB AND FAMILY

Isn't the ability to practice the reason why you went to school? If your family is in California and you want to practice near them eventually, why do you want to take a school acceptance elsewhere?

It is challenging to find a job in a new state as a fresh graduate with no network. The same applies for acquiring a practice. If you did, for lack of options, go to school in a different state than your home state, remember to continue networking within organized dentistry (dental associations, study clubs, and other support groups) in your home state so it becomes easier for you to find an associateship.

If you do end up going to a school that is not in your home state or want to relocate elsewhere after graduation, consider reaching out to dental schools, local dental societies, and study clubs in your destination city while still in school. Make it a point to meet people and network as much as you can over the break. Look for internships or shadowing opportunities to take up during your breaks. All these little things will help you connect with more people and build authentic relationships.

Getting Licensed

Practicing dentistry in the US, like in other countries, requires getting a dental license after graduation. Licensure is a long and expensive process that involves several exams and, at the time of this writing, a clinical board examination. There are five types of clinical board examinations: Council of Interstate Testing Agencies (CITA), Central Regional Dental Testing Services, Inc. (CRDTS), The Commission for Dental Competency Assessments, Southern Regional Testing Agency, Inc (SRTA), and Western Regional Examining Board (WREB) that you can take in the last few months of dental school prior to graduation. Each type of Board gives you the ability to apply for licensure in different states of the US. If you're one of the lucky few who have multiple dental school acceptances, pick carefully so you save yourself the stress of trying to coordinate a board examination in another state.

Some schools allow you to take the Board examination on-site, while others require you to fly to another city and bring patients with you. This quickly adds to costs and overall anxiety. Make the right decision about where you want to go to school.

Note: Ensuring that you follow all the requirements of your state by sitting for the right Board examination is your responsi-bility. Schools can only offer guidance. Requirements also change often, so make sure to remain in touch with your home state licensing board throughout your final year.

BUYING A PRACTICE

If you're looking to own a practice right after school, investigate dental-specific demographics as early as possible, maybe even while applying to dental schools. This will give you an amazing head start. Our most successful peers are those who planned ahead and used their time wisely. While I was enjoying my holidays back in Dubai, some of my colleagues in dental school were taking up internships at private offices and looking for practices to acquire. One dental student did demographic testing while in his second year of dental school. As a result, he had a wonderful practice to buy within months of graduation.

COLLABORATION

I went to a school where we were integrated into a class full of domestic students. Many international students will never have this experience, but for me, it was one of the reasons I chose my school. I wanted to be in a collaborative environment and learn and grow with my domestic colleagues. If you have an opportunity to go to a school like this, I'd highly encourage it. My school and integrated class is the way I met my best friend and co-founder of the New Dentist Business Club. You will get exposed to different views and learn about classmates from different parts of the state and country. That said, you may not have some unique advantages, such as a tailor-made program for international students or networking opportunities among employers who frequently sponsor work visas, that non-integrated programs in other schools get. Pick your battle.

8

LIFE IN SCHOOL AS A FTD

You got an acceptance, took a loan (or did not), and made it into school. Yay!

Life in school goes by quickly. You get busy getting to know your classmates, finishing requirements, and are soon seeing patients. Here are a few things that might make life easier for you.

IMPROVE YOUR COMMUNICATION AND LEADERSHIP SKILLS

Although many of us grew up speaking English, the truth is that American English, with its diversity of accents, is very different from what we were accustomed to back home. If you are shy about raising your hand in class, consider joining a local Toastmasters Club or taking classes in Improv Comedy. Take every opportunity to build more confidence, participate in class, and stand out.

RETAIN WHAT MAKES YOU DIFFERENT

Contrary to what most people think, retain what makes you different. Mainly, continue speaking your language fluently and build a community outside of school where you can connect with people who speak the same language as you. During dental school, I volunteered with the dental van at the local gurudwara (holy place of worship for Sikh's and followers of Guru Nanak).

I became the resident translator and quickly became everyone's favorite dental student at the gurudwara. Years later, after I grad-uated, I continued serving the community at my gurudwara as their lead dentist. This work gave me a lot of satisfaction, and the community became my home away from home. Consider also volunteering at your dental school as a translator in your language.

Build Cultural Competency

Chances are that the city in which your school is based is home to several immigrant communities. Find out who these people are and try to understand their cultures better. Learn how healthcare is practiced in their communities and begin to empathize with their backgrounds. *Pulling Wisdom,* a book written by Dr. Cathy Hung, is a great way to learn different cultural competency skills as a healthcare provider.

Take More CE (Continuing Education) As A Student

One of the greatest advantages of being a student is the ability to benefit from student discounts. Most courses charge dental students peanuts compared to even new dentists. Students also have a wonderful opportunity to get invited as guests to study clubs and dental society meetings for free or at a reduced cost. Use these opportunities to network with new dentists, learn what you love in dentistry and what you want to focus on in the future. Some of these associations may lead you to your future job. One of the specialists I met via a support group helped me find an associateship when I was moving to the Bay Area. Yes, people are *that* nice!

Build A Network

Slowly but surely, build a network of supporters, advisors, and mentors around yourself. Build authentic relationships with teachers and your classmates. One of my closest friends from dental school was a student in the traditional DDS batch. We were tight friends in school and are now business partners. We run a nonprofit together, New Dentist Business Club, where we teach new dentists and den-tal students about the business side of dentistry. This could be you, too.

Take Up Leadership Opportunities

Depending on your school, ASDA may or may not be active. Consider joining them if they are active. Consider volunteering with the Student Council or joining the local dental society and attending their monthly meetings. Why? It helps build expo-sure, and you could connect with potential employers and work opportunities.

Keep Educating Yourself

Listen to dental podcasts and read books about the busi-ness side of dentistry. After long dreary nights being stuck in the prost-hodontics sim lab, I'd listen to some of my favorite podcasts on the way home and feel encouraged by the positivity outside of a student dental clinic. It helped keep things in perspective. More importantly, get some thick skin while you're in dental school. There may be professors who discourage you, patients who are mean, and times when you think to yourself, *Why did I sign up for this a second time?* Uplifting podcasts, books, and mentors will help you through the tough times.

Put Your Name On Every Employment Listserv

Do it as soon as you can—and as early as possible. It can even be as early as a year before graduation. Why? Most of you reading this are immigrants and are already privy to the specific details required by your visa status. Essentially, you need to find a job and visa sponsor within x number of months upon graduation. You don't have much time to waste after graduation. So, use your time in school well. Most schools have alumni groups and listservs that put up practice buying or associate opportunities.

Work On Your Resume

Make sure to work on your resume and have it checked by mul-tiple people at your school. Most schools have counselors who can look through your resume and point out errors. Suffice it to say that leadership positions and publications are always looked at in a positive light.

Buy A Second Set Of Loupes

Everything becomes expensive as soon as you have a DDS/DMD behind your name. Buy a second set of loupes while you're in dental school and take advantage of that student discount.

Attend All "Lunch And Learns" And ASDA-Held Events At Your School

At my school, we were invited to several "lunch and learns" from dental corporations, community health centers, group practices—all trying to hire future dentists. We even heard from banks, dental labs, accountants, lawyers, etc., who wanted to work with dental students. If you're part of ASDA, advocate for more diverse speakers, nonprofits, and dental study clubs to come speak to your class and learn the benefits of joining these micro-communities.

Find Mentors

Having a supportive network of friends and colleagues to rely on will benefit you like nothing else. Finding mentors takes time and in most cases, several years. Mentors can be very important for your career advancement. They can nominate you for awards, advocate for your promotion, help you find a job in a new city, and so much more. That said, learn the respectful way of asking people for help. Although social media has made it easy to reach out to others, it does not mean we should ask a parade of ques-tions to strangers. Be mindful of everyone's time and availability.

TIP: If you're curious about a potential mentor, ask for their business card at a conference. Text them the following day, always starting with how their conversation made you feel, thanking them for their time, and then asking if they would be open to coffee or lunch one day for you to hear more about their experiences. Most people would love to be taken out for lunch and asked about their lives. This is a great conversation starter.

9

WORK OPPORTUNITIES AFTER SCHOOL

You're here and *finally* done with dental school! What now? What options are ahead of you?

One of the biggest issues I faced while preparing for gradu-ation is the lack of enough alumni with whom to discuss potential jobs. I was on a student visa with a one-year OPT (Optional Practical Training) ahead of me. Not many dentists out there are willing to sponsor an H1-B (temporary nonimmi-grant work visa) for a foreign- trained dentist. For more details on H1-B and immigration, skip ahead to read the Interview with Dr. Matthew Ho, a fellow graduate of the UW-IDDS program.

As a foreign-trained dentist, I wanted to talk to people who had been through the same situation as me. At the time, UW had a class size of only eight. Our program was newer and did not have a robust IDDS alumni network yet. There were only a handful of graduates in the past who needed a visa sponsor, and I happened to be one of them.

This is in sharp contrast to students who graduate from a class size of 40–100 international students. Such classes can lean on each other for support and have an alumni network to seek help from.

TIP: If you are in a small international class, it becomes more important for you to advocate for yourself. If you don't speak up, nobody else will. Ask for immigration help from your school. Raise your hand and ask visa related questions to speakers at your school. If you are unable to get resources to guide you during your time as a student, make sure to give back your time later once you're a practicing dentist.

WHY THINK ABOUT WORK OPPORTUNITIES EVEN BEFORE YOU APPLY TO SCHOOLS?

As of this writing, I am aware of several colleagues who are getting their work visas sponsored by employers who are providing them with a below-average work environment. Coupled with poor pay, long commute times, and an uneven mix of patients, there is little opportunity for professional growth for some colleagues. A colleague once told me, "It would've been better if I'd stayed in India and expanded my dad's existing clinic. The struggle to get here is not worth it. I wish I'd considered more seriously the problems with a lottery-based visa and the decade-long wait for a green card."

That said, there's a variety of work options after dental school. Here, we will discuss only the most common.

Jobs here are called associateships. You could have an associ-ateship at a private practice (a small dental clinic privately owned by a dentist), corporate practice (dental support organizations that run several practices that may or may not be owned by a dentist), or go into community health (dental clinics run by the government, often located in rural or underserved areas). You could go into specialty training, also known as 'residencies' after a DDS too. For more info on residency programs, skip ahead to Chapter 10.

PRIVATE PRACTICE ASSOCIATESHIPS

Most of my classmates who went to work with private practice dentists had to work at at least two offices during the week because many of those dentists had only two- or three-day openings. I too practice at a private practice currently.

I work clinically for only a few days and have chosen not to take a second associateship. This could be you as well. My reasons for that are based on work -life balance and compensation received. Most associates like me, who earn on commission, may not need to take a second job if they have a busy schedule of patients daily. However, if you are a new graduate, you will ini-tially have a slower schedule and not be as busy. This may mean that you may need to take two or three such part-time jobs to earn enough. Keep this in mind.

In the US, dental insurance is a big industry. Many patients have dental insurance and will want to rightfully, utilize it at their dental office. Dental insurance reimbursement rates tend to be better at private offices. Most private offices also take fewer insurance plans and see many fee-for-service (cash paying) patients. This directly translates to fewer patients on your schedule but more value for each procedure. Essentially, if you choose to be in private practice long term, you will likely be working fewer days and hours to make the same as your friends in corporate dentistry.

Note: It is imperative to mention here that many private practices will not be comfortable sponsoring a work visa for you. It is a lot of paperwork for any dentist to prepare. Find a practice owner who is well versed with the nitty gritty of the complicated immigration system in the US and has been through the process with another associate before.

Helpful questions to consider asking during an interview for any associateship:

1. Ask what the previous associate on average made (took home) or their production so you get an accurate estimate of what income you will draw. In a busy office, you never need to worry about pay. In newer offices or during slow months (summer), you do. In those cases, some employers offer a daily minimum to keep you afloat.

2. Remember to negotiate your pay based on the market you are in. Ask your colleagues or your school for advice about what the market pay for a recent graduate in your area is. Unless you bring a different set of skills to the table, like implants or sedation, the pay you are offered is the same as that given to any other fresh grad with a DDS. Do not settle for less than market pay. For another perspective on why it is crucial to negotiate, skip to Chapter 11.

3. Ask how many assistants will be working specifically with you; having two assistants usually means you will be busy.

4. Ask how many days and hours you'll be working, how many patients you are expected to see on any given day, and is there room for procedure in addition to the practice? For example, can you start doing surgical extractions and implant placements (if that's what you love to do)?

5. A lot of associates put value on mentorship but what I've found is that mentorship becomes available to you only if you seek it. There are always ways to find it, no matter which associateship you are in. Don't stress about having your boss be your mentor; in most cases, that is not pos-sible or likely.

6. Some private offices may not want to hire you if you're on a visa. They think of it as an invest-ment with an unpredictable return. What if you don't get the lottery work visa next year? What if you must leave the country for some reason and never come back? How complicated does hiring a foreigner have to be? Turns out, very. I have personally been denied a few associateships for this very reason.

7. Be open to seeking counsel from an immigration attorney if you have questions about your visa status and maintaining job security.

8. On your resume, put it in **bold** that you are foreign-trained, and you need sponsorship for a visa.

CORPORATE ASSOCIATESHIPS

There are a ton of corporate dental chains out there, and unfor-tunately, most of them get a bad reputation from dental schools. However, note that many dental students end up working with corporates for the first five years out of school, and a few will work for them throughout their lives.

I worked at two corporate practices soon after graduation. Here is a snapshot of my experience in both:

1. Contrary to what you will hear in school or dental society meetings, nobody planned the treatment of a patient for me. If this ever happens to you, remember that this is illegal. Dentistry is a highly regulated profession in this country, and your license is on the line.

2. The assistants and office managers I worked with during my corporate associateships were some of the nicest, most motivated team members I have ever worked with.

3. Employment contracts are hard to introduce any changes to. I have seen contracts with an exit notice period ranging from three months to nine months. Always have a lawyer read your contract and look out for potential red flags. This is money well spent and will save you heartache down the road.

4. Corporate offices typically have you accept a lot of insur-ance plans, see patients with Medicaid (government spon-sored insurance), and serve a busy community. This number varies greatly, but in some offices, you will see upwards of 40–50 patients a day. This can be great if you're interested in bringing up your speed. However, be wary of burnout. About a year and a half in, I spotted the signs of early burn-out and quit my high-paying, four-day-a-week cor-porate associateship to pursue my current two-day-a-week private practice associateship. I now have more peace of mind, time for other hobbies, and I can take care of my health better. I also found time to finally write this book!

Interview With Matthew Ho, DDS

Note: The following interview details a successful journey from a work visa sponsorship to a permanent residency status. Experience shared and opinions expressed are that of the author alone. It is important for you to consult with an immigration attorney regarding your specific situation and stay abreast of any policy/fee changes.

Interview excerpt from Dr. Matthew Ho, 2018 University of Washington School of Dentistry IDDS (International DDS) graduate

SD: You graduated from UW with a DDS in 2018 and are now in a corporate practice. Are you being sponsored a work visa by your practice? What was the process like?

MH: I was sponsored by my employer for a working visa and green card. At the end of one year of OPT (Optional Practical Training), at about a year and a half out, I got my green card.

As of 2019, the following was the fee schedule in my case for "H1B (nonimmigrant) working visa": $2,000/- for the lawyer working on filing my working visa and a government fee of around $1,800/-. Some people want their cases to be reviewed quicker by USCIS (United States Citizenship & Immigration Services). You can pay extra for that; it's $ 1,400/- for premium processing. Those fees technically need to be paid by H1B visa applicants; however, my employer paid those for me (except the premium processing fee).

There are some fees for applying for an H1B working visa that need to be paid by the employer: an ACWIA fee (American

Competitiveness and Workforce Improvement Act) and a fraud prevention fee. Together it was about $1,300/-.

In 2019, the year I applied, things ran on a lottery basis. Under the regular cap, the limit was 65,000. This means, for that year, only 65,000 people get their H1B visa, and if your educational level is above masters—such as a graduate of the IDDS (International Doctor of Dental Surgery) program like me—the limit extends to 20,000 more seats. This means we get a bigger chance than others.

The only other way to get H1B, if not through a lottery, is to get a job at a university, dental school, or nonprofit.

Timeline: the beginning of the year (between January and February) is preparation time. This is when you must find a lawyer, so make sure your documents are in order.

March to April is when USCIS releases its results based on the lottery.

If your application gets accepted, your OPT will automatically be extended to September 30th, and then your H1-B visa starts on October 1st of that year.

If it doesn't get accepted, your legal status expires 60 days after the expiry date on your OPT. Some people choose to apply for another continuing education program with an F1 student visa or work for a nonprofit or in a university setting if they want to continue staying in America.

People might need to consider the prevailing wage too. This depends on where you are working and what type of job you have. USCIS has set a prevailing wage for the area.

There are two things I'd like to mention here. Once you get your H1-B visa, you must make sure your income matches the prevailing wage. This is necessary for you to comply with the government's expectations.

Also, to apply for H1-B, all applicants need to find a related job; it must be degree-related. You can't work in a restaurant or supermarket, for example. It must be dental-related, such as a research assistant, dental assistant, dentist, etc.

SD: Did you have a lot of options when it came to picking an office to work for that would be willing to sponsor a work visa? What were your other options at the time?

MH: I was introduced to my current job by a perio resident graduate. We knew from before that this employer was willing to sponsor a working visa and green card.

The only other option for me was a corporate office in Puyallup, Washington State, but they did not offer a great salary; the pay was minimum, and I could only get an H1 -B visa. We didn't talk about green card sponsorship during that interview.

My goal at the time was to get a working visa and green card as soon as possible. That's why I took a job in Sequim (remote area), which is quite far from the city of Seattle (and Puyallup).

SD: Did you take student loans to fund your education? Was it a local bank or a bank in your home country? How are you managing to pay off those loans?

MH: I did take loans from my home country, from the govern-ment. I'd say it was a pretty good deal. For the first five years, we have a grace period where we don't have to pay off anything, and then they waive the interest for ten years. I did work in my home country for a few years, so I had some savings from what I made back then to put towards tuition.

Currently, I am putting a certain percentage of my income every month towards paying down my loans.

SD: What advice do you have for FTD graduates looking to get their permanent residency and a good job here?

MH: First, the most important thing is connections; commu-nicate with faculty, schoolmates, graduates; they will offer you jobs, resources, perhaps introduce you to a friend, and maybe they will open a new office and are looking for a new associate.

Dentistry is a closed field. It's not very open, so you must net-work, especially for foreign-trained dentists. You must ask faculty, graduates, and other friends to help you.

In my opinion, the more suburban areas you are in, the more chances you get for a green card. It is very competitive in the city. Why would employers pay an extra fee to hire an FTD in the city rather than a local dentist? They don't have to worry about extra fees, government fees, etc. They don't need financial documents disclosed under inspection when hiring a local dentist.

Finally, you must make sure your income matches the prevailing wage, so find out what the prevailing wage is for your area. Ask your lawyer; they will give you a better idea if you will be okay. You will need that to maintain PR (permanent residency) visa/ status.

For further questions, reach Dr. Matthew Ho directly at qqmat-thewqq@gmail.com

Growing As An Associate

A short note on pay structures: Private offices and corporate offices usually offer you a daily minimum and a percentage of production. 'Production' implies the total $ value of your work for the day. For example, if you placed 5 crowns on Monday, valued at $1000/- each and you make a 30% of production per your employer, you earned $1500/ - for the day (this does not include tax deduction). If you went to work on Tuesday and saw no patients (because they all cancelled or rescheduled), you can still make your minimum pay- whatever was negotiated between you and your employer.

If you go to work in public health, you are most likely paid a set salary- it does not matter what the $ value of your production of the day was, you will always make the same income per month.

Whichever associateship you pick, the hope is for all of you, foreign-trained dentists, to be successful and thriving. Here are a few additional tips to make you love your job.

1. Ask others for feedback. Not just mentors, but colleagues, dental assistants, office managers—everyone. In my second year of associateships, I had a great working relationship with my dental assistant. So, I asked her to begin shad-owing me and give feedback about the way I presented treatment and built case acceptance. At the time of asking, I honestly wasn't sure what she would come up with. Turns out she had a ton of feedback for me, from body language to tone—even the way in which I describe treatment—my anesthesia technique and the way I wedge prior to fillings. She opened my mind to a huge number of gaps, and I have always been grateful for it.

2. Always be intentional. Before signing up for a speaker's lecture or attending a clinical education course, ask your-self, "Will I need this to achieve my goals?" Your time is valuable. It'll be tempting to attend all kinds of courses, even ones that are expensive, but if you keep reminding yourself of your why, you'll be intentional and more mind-ful about your expenses.

3. Don't lose faith in your beliefs; just keep going. Don't doubt yourself, don't look at other people's clinical successes and think, *Why not me?* Heartily congratulate them, feel good about them, and when the time is right, ask them

for feed-back about what you could do to improve. Focus on building those friendships along the way.

Interview With Delphine Jeong, DMD

Note: The following conversation discusses immigration, work visa sponsorship and the struggle behind gaining permanent residency. All opinions expressed herein are that of the author. Please consult with an immigration attorney regarding your specific situation. Remember that policies around immigration are constantly evolving.

This is an interview with Delphine Jeong, DMD, a 2015 gradu-ate of Boston University, Henry M. Goldman School of Dental Medicine.

SD: You graduated from undergrad and dental school in the US and then moved to Canada for work opportunities. What inspired you to make the move?

DJ: I wasn't very happy in the States. I spent four years in Indiana for my undergrad and experienced quite a bit of racism while I was a student. For example, I was once refused a job on the college campus and told, "we are not looking for an Asian to work here."

I tried to fit into American culture. However, things like that were almost daily occurrences, and it was not a good environ-ment for me.

As an international student, I was paying the highest tuition in the US, yet often treated poorly. On the other hand, I remember feeling welcomed whenever I visited Canada, always greeted with, "Welcome to Canada!"

I also loved the novelty of moving to another country. I was born and raised in France, grew up in South Korea, and had finished my education in the US. So, I was ready for something new, a new challenge. My sister also had a Canadian PR, and I wanted the opportunity to be closer to her.

SD: Did you have a lot of options when it came to picking an office that would be willing to sponsor a work visa? What were your other options in 2015? Did you have to work with a lawyer?

DJ: I interviewed at ten to twelve places; most of them were cold calls. I interviewed in person and over the phone, and none of them were interested in providing work visa sponsorship. Then, through the network of familial connections, I met the dentist owner of a small- town practice in Alberta, who eventually became my sponsor and employer.

The other opportunity was in a place far up north called Northwest Territories for a three-year contract. It is a cold and dark place with long winters, zero sunlight, and temperatures around neg-ative 40 or 50 degrees Celsius. I couldn't possibly be locked in for three years, so I chose the option in Alberta.

I worked with a lawyer, converting from visitor status to work permit, and now PR (permanent residency).

The first time that I went through the PR process was without a lawyer, and I got rejected. I applied with a lawyer the second time, and it went well. The work visa cost me between $5,000-8,000/-, and permanent residency cost $5,000/- (Canadian dollars).

SD: How well do you think your school prepared you for life after DDS/DMD as a foreign-trained dentist?

DJ: It was our job to find work opportunities. It was our job to reach out to clinics and find employment. The school does not prepare you for that.

SD: What would be your advice to future graduates?

DJ: Use your connections (you'll have more chances of finding a sponsor) and be prepared.

You'll find many sponsors in remote areas. I went there without knowing exactly what I was getting myself into and ended up feeling completely alone in a small town. I got there in the winter and suffered for three years from depression.

If you can build your network and connections prior to moving, especially so you have a support system, that'll be better.

When you are getting sponsored, try to read the person who is sponsoring you. Do not take the first opportunity you get. Find out what the owner doctor is like, what their reputation is like in the community, and ask yourself, "Will this person treat me well and pay me fairly?"

Read your contract thoroughly. Before signing anything, review it, know what the conditions are, and what is entailed. If they don't have a contract, make certain to have one prepared.

Establish boundaries, both legally and personally, before you even start the job.

Do not rush into it, do not be in a desperate position, have confidence that you have a great set of skills, and approach it in that sense. Don't be desperate about taking whatever comes along. Remember that when someone sponsors you, it must be a win-win situation.

I believe that if you stay grounded and centered, you will attract the right sponsors.

You can connect directly with Dr. Jeong at delsjeong@gmail.com

Practice Ownership

Many of you will choose to dive into practice ownership as soon as possible. Practice ownership can be a very fulfilling yet stressful experience. It is also the best way to gain financial freedom early in your career and build the work-life balance you want.

Here is what Ketan Jumani, DDS, MSD, MPH, says about building an authentic brand around his work as a pediatric dental practice owner in Sammamish, WA state.

> Be genuine, honest, and do good work. When you are start-ing a practice and want to build your brand, it is important to do exceptional work and to know what your limits are. As a specialist, the buck ends with you, and this is the only way your referral sources will trust you.

> You cannot afford to have many screwups; we live in a very litigious society. Our society is also, sadly, very review driven. So, always try to focus on doing good work and being kind and honest.

> In my practice, I don't leave any part of the patient experi-ence to chance. I have streamlined systems in place. There's a thought that goes behind everything. For example, what show is playing on Netflix when a certain family comes in, who is greeting a specific patient, who's going to check in with the patient. Ensuring patients have a smooth and seamless experience is what will ultimately make you successful. For the most part, everyone is doing good dentistry. It's the little things that separate you from the dentist down the street.

Ketan also mentions the importance of networking as a prac-ticing pediatric dentist in the community:

> When you're new in a city, you must introduce yourself, take colleagues out to lunch. Doing those working lunches has gone a long way in helping me build my brand. What

is also important is being kind, genuine, conscientious, and com-passionate. I want to be known as the dentist who will always do the right thing.

Trust doesn't come overnight. It takes time. Being kind and honest is what builds trust. I am Indian and speak different languages; I own it and am proud of it. But I am also Ameri-can. Learning about US culture, traditions, holidays, current events, news, etc., has helped me build trust with my patients and connect with my community.

You can connect directly with Dr. Jumani by emailing him at ketan.jumani@gmail.com

10

RESIDENCY PROGRAMS

A lot of foreign-trained dentists do not want to go through a DDS to practice in the US. They want to go into specialty programs or residencies directly. Here is an interview with Dr. Manali Vora, who is a current periodontics resident at University of Connecticut.

SD: You worked for two years as a postdoc after completing your MPH and are now pursuing your dream goal of perio residency. Was it challenging to find schools willing to take foreign-trained dentists as residents?

MV: This is a great question. Taking the step towards doing a perio residency was not easy. All program directors are very welcoming and invite questions from applicants. They are also very honest. While doing my postdoc at UCSF, I met with a lot of program directors and asked them all what they were looking for in an applicant and what I should be doing to improve my candidacy. Many of them told me the same thing—not having any US clinical experience will be a cause of concern.

Schools are looking for students who will not have any trouble getting used to the rigorous clinical pace of residency life. So yes,

I was nervous about applying to programs, and I'll be honest that I did not get a lot of interviews. The interviews I did get, how-ever, were very nice, and I was fortunate enough to be matched at my favorite program.

Most residencies welcome applicants of a foreign-trained back-ground, but they like you to have clinical experience in the US. Many schools don't even require you to give your NBDE. However, because competition is tough, you, as a foreign -trained dentist, need to do a lot more and have a more packed resume compared to the typical US or Canadian-trained dentist.

Coming to the US as a resident straight after dental school from another country is a lot harder because of all these factors.

SD: How would a dentist with a BDS (Bachelor of Dental Surgery) from another part of the world prepare for applying to residency programs in the US?

MV: If you are interested in a residency program, you should first go to the PASS (Postdoctoral Application Support Service) website and look at its resources.

Most people applying to post-grad programs in India, for example, are open to multiple branches. An important distinction to make here is that in the US, you apply to only one branch. You must show serious intention towards one specific branch (ex: perio) and demonstrate why you want to do the program. Commitment is what all programs are looking for.

Start with the PASS website, look at all the schools participating, then study all the school websites and look at their prerequisites. Some schools won't accept your application unless you have a green card or are a US citizen. However, you are not limited. There are plenty of programs that will accept you despite your immigration status. Have a checklist of schools; get organized.

I personally applied to about fifteen programs. If you're not in the US and are not familiar with the system, it does get tough. You must time yourself to ensure your application is turned in early and is complete.

There are also externship opportunities at many schools. You can shadow at a program you are interested in for a few days to a week. This helps you network, understand how the application system works, and meet residents.

I am serious here; I took two years to simply understand the sys-tem and properly apply to PASS. I would recommend every-one start early and get organized.

SD: Do you know how many people applied for and inter-viewed at your program?

MV: Twenty people were interviewed, and two were accepted. I am not completely sure how many people applied; I am guessing there were at least a couple hundred.

I interviewed only in smaller programs, which was a personal preference. The odds of you matching at your favorite program are not too high, so give yourself plenty of time to get into the program you want to be in.

SD: Do you have tips for interviews?

Interviews are relatively relaxed. The faculty want to know who you are as a person. They might ask you stuff about your resume, but mostly, they want to know if you'd be a good fit for the program.

Answer questions well, practice if you must, and be genuine.

Keep up with the program, learn what makes it unique, learn about different faculty members and their research work, and ask questions during your interview. Remember, you are inter-viewing them too.

These are day-long interviews from 8 a.m. to 5 p.m. and include an office tour, faculty interview, and a social component where you are taken out for lunch and drinks with the residents. Be relaxed and be yourself.

SD: Applications, travel, and externship opportunities sound expensive. How did you finance your journey to and through residency?

MV: I was working for a few years and was saving up for applications.

There is tuition mentioned very clearly on every program web-site. Be realistic and ask yourself, "Can I afford this?" Include previous years' fees for the cost of living, books, and food. Some programs are extremely expensive; keep this in mind when you apply. Once you match a program, you must pay up. A matching process means you get one acceptance and not multiple.

On that note, there's a limit to how much you can borrow from banks too.

If your fees are too high, that may become a problem. All those things should work in sync. Once you match, you can always apply for a private loan. I had to have a US citizen cosign my education loan. Having someone cosign your loan is a big deal. They are acting like your guarantee, and they need to have a good credit score and trust you completely.

Financing is tricky but don't let that be the reason you don't apply for higher education. Remember that the money is an investment in yourself. You will be able to pay off your student loans.

You could also get private loans from US banks or take a loan from whichever country you come from. If you've just finished dental school in your home country, you may or may not qualify for a big loan. It will be based on what your family (or parents) can afford. Educational loans from your home country typically require a collateral. Non-collateral loans are usually very small and don't cover US tuition.

SD: Can you talk a little about repayment plans after finishing up a residency?

MV: Yes, there is something called an income repayment plan. You can choose to repay your US loan right after school or per-haps defer it for six months after graduation. Most loans you will be able to pay back in ten to fifteen years. You may have to live like a student for at least four or five years after graduation. It is worth it, though.

* * *

Ketan Jumani, DDS, MPH, MSD, completed a pediatric resi-dency at UW after his DDS program there. He gives further tips on building a competitive portfolio as a candidate for residency:

> Pediatrics, like OMFS and perio, is an incredibly competitive program to get into. People say grades don't matter, but they do matter. How else would you differentiate people when all candidates have stellar resumes?
>
> Having a good GPA, class rank, shadowing other pediatric programs, doing electives in pediatrics, and significant previ-ous work experience matters. I also did a lot of research

in the department of orthodontics during my time in dental school. Ultimately, I think my MPH also played a critical role in my acceptance.

For more information on residency programs, here is the link to the PASS website: https://www.adea.org/pass/

Several international students apply directly to residency programs, without having been through a traditional advanced standing program. Know, however, that there is a key factor that affects their work opportunities after graduation.

Graduates of several residency programs, even after receiving Board licensure, may be restricted to only certain states for their practice. A dentist with a DDS typically does not have such restrictions, as long as they comply with Board requirements of their target state. On the other hand, some residency pro-gram graduates (periodontics, endodontics, AEGD- Advanced Education in General Dentistry, etc.) may have to wait several years (completing a certain number of hours of practice) before moving to another state to work. Others may only have the option to take up academic positions at a university if they wish to move to another state after their program.

TIP: When choosing a residency program to go to, take some time to read and understand requirements of licensure in your target state. Don't hesitate to call the state Board and ask questions. Mention that you are an international student and do not have a DDS when you do so.

11

PRACTICING IN CANADA

Kanika Sabhlok, DDS, one of my classmates from Manipal University, India, now practices in Canada. She answered commonly asked questions about the licensure process in Canada, job opportunities, and gave advice to those interested in moving there.

Note: We had the following conversation in 2020-2021. Licensing routes and immigration policies may have changed by the time you read this. Stay updated on changes via links listed in 'Further Resources'.

SD: You completed a DDS at UCLA and now practice in Canada. Did you consider practicing in Canada without going through the US-DDS route? If yes, what does that process look like?

KS: Honestly, my answer to this question is yes and no. I always wanted to do a DDS, and after my BDS in India, I wanted to get those two years of DDS in to learn how dentistry is practiced in North America. I wanted to learn not only the clinical side but also medico-legal aspects and patient management.

I did investigate direct licensing in Canada and took the first part of the exam. However, before I could finish that route, I got accepted at UCLA for a DDS. Therefore, I went ahead with my plans for a DDS. Perhaps if I hadn't gotten accepted that year, I would've considered getting licensed directly.

SD: What do you mean by getting licensed directly? What are the steps for that to happen?

KS: Before I explain any further, look up this link: https://ndeb-bned.ca/en/requirements. This page explains the three options, one for graduates from an accredited program in the US and Canada like myself and the other two are for direct licensing, for being able to practice dentistry in Canada.

The first column is what I went through. I went through an accred-ited program in the US (others could do it here in Canada) and then took my OSCE (Objective Structured Clinical Examination) and written exams, got my certification, and later my provincial license.

The OSCE or multiple -choice questions are always challenging. However, if you put in a few months of independent study while you're still in your accredited program, you can pass it on your first attempt, like I did. As of 2020, the pass rate for graduates in 2020 was 86 percent in the written examination and 94 percent in OSCE.

Once NDEB (National Dental Examination Board of Canada) gives you a certificate saying you've passed the exam, you can then apply to a specific province for getting your license.

Unlike in the US, where different states have a different board exam, here in Canada, we have one national exam. Once you pass that exam, you only seek permission from a specific province to be able to practice there.

SD: How do foreign-trained dentists get licensed to practice in Canada?

KS: If you don't go through an accredited program like I did, you have two other options. One is for general practitioners, and the other is for specialists.

For general practitioners, you go through an NDEB equivalency process. In this process, there are three exams you take: AFK (Assessment of Fundamental Knowledge), ACJ (Assessment of Clinical Judgement), and ACS (Assessment of Clinical Skills).

The AFK exam, which is also multiple-choice, is very similar to the NDEB written exam I took after my DDS at UCLA. There are two ways you can go from here. You can either get a very competitive score and gain admission into a Canadian school for a DDS program or get a passing score and proceed with the other two exams: ACJ and ACS.

ACS is a lot like the bench tests we give in the US.

ACJ is an in-person interview, where they give you real-life patient scenarios, such as x-rays, models, reports, etc., and deter-mine your clinical judgment to see if it is on par with North American-trained dentists. Most foreign-trained dentists, to my knowledge, struggle with these two exams: ACS and ACJ.

The overall percentage of people who pass those last two exams is much lower. In the equivalency process in 2021, the pass rate of candidates giving the ACS was 66 percent, and ACJ was 62 percent.

The process for specialists (i.e., graduates of ortho, perio, etc.) from other countries is slightly different from those of us general dentists. You take a theory exam, the DSCKE (Dental Specialty Core Knowledge Examination), for your specialty. This score is used by the dental schools in Canada to determine your eligibil-ity into the DSAPT (Dental Specialty Assessment and Training Programs), wherein you spend one to two years at a school in an accredited program and only then can practice as a specialist in Canada.

SD: Do you have any recommendations for candidates looking to prepare for direct licensing?

KS: In every major city, there are courses to prepare FTDs for these exams. I would recommend interested candidates do their research prior to signing up for them as these courses can cost a pretty penny. None of these are endorsed by the NDEB. You should also be prepared to travel to specific cities within Canada for these courses and live in the area for a few months to prepare.

TIP: Do your research, network with friends, and ask around for recommendations about the right course. Make sure to budget not only for your course but also for living and traveling expenses.

SD: What is the concept of reciprocity in Canada when it comes to licensure? Can you explain it?

KS: If you've graduated with a dental degree from certain countries (e.g., the US, Ireland, New Zealand, Australia), you're considered to have completed an accredited program in Canada. This means that graduates from these countries get to go directly through the first column route that I did.

SD: What are the different kinds of practice opportunities available to FTDs?

KS: First things first, to practice in Canada, you cannot be on a work permit like in the US. You need to have a permanent residency or citizenship. To write any of the exams (AFK, ACJ, or ACS), you don't need your PR; however, for licensure, you do need it in place.

A lot of foreign-trained dentists who have graduated from an accredited program in the US or Canada qualify for an express PR. It is not just for dentists; a lot of other professionals benefit from this program as well—medicine, IT, etc. In the past year (2020), we have had a net influx of many such professionals from the US to Canada.

The pay offered to dentists is 30–40 percent of production or collection unless you have abilities like re- treatment of endo and implants, sedation, etc., in which case you can negotiate higher. The difference between production or collection is not much because most practices in Canada are fee-for-service, and collection rates are quite high. Practices may do direct billing, but the concept of in-network providers from insurance companies is not common here, like in the US.

Once you have a license, look for a job far and wide. Look online, in local dental societies, and on dental school websites. Make sure you are a good fit for the office and vice versa. Mentorship was important to me when I first graduated and so was working for people who have good systems in place and practice ethical dentistry. It may take you a few positions to find a practice you thrive in, so don't be discouraged. Do not compromise on your morals; you worked hard to get your license, no matter what route you took. So, remember, your license is your most valuable asset.

Many fresh graduates choose to practice in a rural setting for six months or more to get exposed to different dental procedures and obtain relatively higher pay due to there being a scarcity of dentists.

Lastly, you can also work for the city in public health. You are offered a starting salary and get some benefits in health and retirement plans.

SD: Can you talk a little about the number of schools in Canada, how many seats there are on average, and what spe-cialty training looks like?

KS:

1. There are only ten dental schools in Canada. Needless to say, getting into a DDS program or specialty is very competitive. Many dentists go to the US to get specialty training for this reason.

2. Schools have a mix of seat numbers. For example, some schools (like University of Toronto and Western) have approximately twenty seats for advanced standing for FTDs. Other schools may have less or none.

3. We don't have any private schools here in Canada, which is again why seats are fewer and competition is tough.

12

FINAL WORDS OF WISDOM

This book was going to remain in my google drive forever had it not been for a few mentors who encouraged me to publish. The reason I share this with you is because if you have just taken the time to read this book in its entirety, you already have it in you to make your dream of getting into dental school come true. You have the fortitude and passion. You are already *Persevering*.

A lot of people lose hope and abandon their dreams of prac-ticing dentistry in the US mid-way through their journey. While it is okay to pivot and change your dreams often, if you've already done the work of reading this book, applying to schools, even gone on a few interviews, you owe it to yourself now to com-plete the process and get into school. Believe me, it will happen.

Like I've said throughout the book; it is only a matter of *time*. See you on the other side!

Below is a collection of final thoughts and advice gathered from a few of the dentists and students who were interviewed for this book.

Nayanika Sanga, DDS, MPH, on advice for students who have been through a few rejections and multiple cycle attempts:

Remember, this is it. This is your toughest phase, and it is as tough as it is going to get. Hang in there and trust the pro-cess. Work on believing in yourself because it is all worth it in the end. Remind yourself that you have the training and the skill set for this, and you will most certainly prevail.

You can reach Dr. Sanga for further advice at sanga.nayanika@gmail.com

Manali Vora, MPH, has advice on keeping your cool during a challenging application process and staying organized:

Everything before matching felt like pure torture. However, matching into UConn made all of it feel worth it.

Don't underestimate your competition. Recognize that you are competing with people who have completely different pro-files. Many of them are DDS applicants with a ton of leader-ship skills, and some are right out of school. Waiting between the application and matching phase is truly nerve-wracking. But keep going. Have patience and hang in there.

The whole process can be strenuous and requires a long time commitment. The process is not that fun, as it is packed with self-doubt. I remember meeting all these amazing people and asking myself, "Why would a school choose me?" Don't let the negativity get to you, though. Just keep your head down, do the work, and give it your best.

Kanika Sabhlok, DDS, provides practical tips for FTDs moving to Canada:

One, before you decide to move here, figure out your finances and come up with a plan. I know a few FTDs who took a long time to finish their journey because they realized, as they were in the middle of the process, how expensive it could be. Plan, plan, plan!

Two, quality of life is very important. Know that if you work as a DDS in more saturated areas in a competitive market, you may make less but work longer hours—like the US.

Three, getting a loan here is doable with a good guarantor once you've been accepted to an accredited program.

Four, some foreign-trained dentists are against the two years of schooling. Don't be too quick to eliminate that route. You learn a lot in those two years; apart from growing clinically, you learn expectations for record-keeping and understand the medico-legal aspects of our profession to practice in North America.

And last, the direct licensing program is not here to replace an education. If you go that route, remember to also learn how to identify a good practice from an unfavorable one, as well as how to manage your practice and negotiate your pay."

You can reach Dr. Sabhlok for further information at ksabhlok@gmail.com

ACKNOWLEDGEMENTS

"It takes a village."

There are a lot of people without whom this book and my professional journey thus far would have remained a distant dream. I'd like to thank my parents, who have always been the strongest supporters any kid could ask for. I know for a fact that going through school rejections one after the other hurt them more than it did me. Mom and dad, I want to thank you both for believing in me, being patient and letting me stumble, hustle, and pave my own way. It would not have been possible without your unconditional support and kindness. I love you guys so much.

I want to thank my sister, Sonali and brother-in-law, Abhijit dada. I'll never forget all the times Abhijit dada drove me to the airport for interviews and to bench prep classes in Milpitas. You guys even flew down with me to my first interview in Colorado. My three-year journey to dental school would have been ridden with a hundred more obstacles had you two not been around. You kept me positive, happy, and well fed. I love and appreciate you both more than you can imagine.

Special thanks to Bina Tai and Vikram Dada for housing me for two whole months in 2013 when I was writing my NBDE Part I and shadowing a local dentist. Thank you for being such gracious hosts. It's because of family like you'll that I am where I am today- you guys are the best!!

I am nothing without my friends and colleagues, many of whom were interviewed for this book. Kanika, apart from being a role model, I hope you know how much your advice impacted me during the early days when I was still struggling with rejections. Thanks for being who you are and for contributing to the Bonus Chapter about practicing in Canada. Ketan, Matthew, Dhara, and Dr. Chan, the IDDS program at the University of Washington is special because of people like you. Thank you for contributing to this book and for supporting the program the way you do. Manali, I am so proud of all that you've accomplished since the time we have known each other. We first met in Seattle, when I was a D4, and you were finishing your MPH. You are now in your residency, and I'm a practicing dentist, how time has flown. And our friendship continues to grow. I am so excited for your future and very grateful for your contribution about residency programs in this book. Nayanika, our fateful meet-ing when you interviewed at the UW has had so many wonderful ripple effects. Our meeting proves that foreign-trained dentists can be each other's biggest support systems and that we should continue thinking of colleagues as friends, not competition. Thank you for getting interviewed for this book. Last but not the least, Delphine, I am so grateful to have gotten to know you via the Creative Collective, and I remain fascinated by your degree of introspection. I hope to continue learning from you for years to come. Thanks for your honest take on the realities of immigration in this book. It is an important perspective many of us need to have prior to embarking on this journey. Thank you also to several students and dentists, including Drs. Andy Tawfik and Smita Kumar, for adding their perspective to Chapter 3 on schools. Having an in-depth understanding of what we are getting ourselves into when we reply 'accept' to a school's offer, is so important.

Books like this take many hours of editing, proofreading, designing, and back and forth emailing. I'd like to thank my editorial and publishing team at JETLAUNCH for spending much time reviewing, editing, and designing this book. Chris, Laura, John and Teri, thank you for being patient with me; you have been such a pleasure to work with. You have made my first book writing experience very pleasant and memorable.

Special thanks to the incredible faculty I've had the plea-sure of learning from. Not only were these individuals great teach-ers, they were also compassionate colleagues. I'd like to thank Dr. RamPrasad Vasthare for being one of the nicest teachers in Manipal. Dr. Vasthare, not only did you write glowing letters of recommendation for me, and proofread our research papers mul-tiple times, you continued to support me even after grad-uation. I have appreciated your mentorship over the years and hope every dental student has a teacher like you in their lives. Dr. Richard Smith, your support and guidance during my time at UCSF was invaluable. I firmly believe our research work together and your mentorship helped me get accepted into dental school. Dr. Avina Paranjpe, your advocacy lends an important lens to our strong IDDS program at the University of Washington. You are a skilled teacher, and I am grateful that our program has you at its forefront. We appreciate you more than you know.

I'd also like to thank Dr. Cathy Hung. I first got to know of you, Dr. Hung, because of your book, *Pulling Wisdom*. Little did I realize that you would be so approachable and would one day become my coach. Thanks for advocating for me and being a pil-lar of strength and wisdom for me. I have so much more to learn from you and I am grateful that fate has brought you into my life. Much thanks also to dear friend, Dr. Diana Harris, who was the first to get excited about my book, insisting she read it, and gave meaningful feedback and much needed mentorship, in making this book possible. Thanks, Diana for the incredible human you are. Your contribution has been invaluable.

Finally, I'd also like to thank Dr. Pai, Dean of Manipal College of Dental Sciences (MCODS) Manipal, who took the time to read the manuscript in its entirety, give feedback and write an Introduction. Thanks Dr. Pai, for being an incredible teacher and for making MCODS Manipal, the wonderful educational institution that it is!

Is any book complete without acknowledging a spouse? Bhushan, where should I even begin? We met when I was in my 3rd year of application cycles, a few weeks before my interview at University of Washington. I was supposed to be stressed and anxious at the time; I was in my 3rd cycle of interviews, after all. However, having you around kept stress at bay and filled me with happy memories instead. Within a few months of accepting UW's offer, you followed me to Seattle so we could work on our relationship together. The rest is history. You are the best friend a girl could ask for. You have been there with me through gradu-ation, numerous associateships, and many side hustles. You have helped me stay calm and always have the best advice to offer. I love you and am grateful that I get to spend every single day with you, for the rest of my life. Also, thank you for doing the dishes, putting away the laundry, and cooking hot meals for me while I was writing this book. I love you.

FURTHER RESOURCES

1. ADEA, American Dental Education Association. All the schools participating in CAAPID have requirements and other details mentioned on ADEA. They host several webi-nars throughout the year, of specific interest to FTDs. Consider signing up for their webinars and reaching out to them for questions. They also have an active presence on YouTube where many of the recorded webinars are posted. Find them at adea.org

2. ADA, American Dental Association. The website itself has several resources for International Dentists. There are also weekly newsletters such as ADA Morning Huddle and New Dentist Now that often carry articles of interest to foreign-trained dentists. American Dental Association also maintains an updated list of all schools that accept foreign-trained dentists, whether they participate in CAAPID or not. American Student Dental Association accepts international dentists as members, even if you are not a dental student in the US yet. Find more information at ada.org

3. Student Doctor Network, the OG. This website carries a wealth of knowledge in its threads, dating all the way back to 1999. It's a nonprofit, and it is what many of us, interviewed in this book, would spend days and nights crawling back before the advent of Facebook, Whatsapp, and Instagram. Studying interview related details on this

website will give you a very clear idea of what schools are looking for. Access it at studentdoctor.net

4. Individual school websites. CAAPID is just half the work. The real work begins on school websites. Every school website provides details on requirements that may change from one year to the next. Chapter 3 is just an overview of requirements as of the year 2021, consider re-evaluating after visiting the individual school website. Stay in touch with the program coordinator to ensure all your documents have been received. Follow up is key.

5. This book only touched the tip of the iceberg when it comes to getting licensed in Canada. Head to https://ndeb-bned. ca for more information.

6. For an updated list of coaches and professionals who can help you build communication skills and provide you with interview day tips, head to my website www.sampadadesh-pandedds.com and search for "coach."

7. To have me come present at your school, dental society, or study club, please contact me via my website to receive a speaker's packet and more details.

ABOUT THE AUTHOR

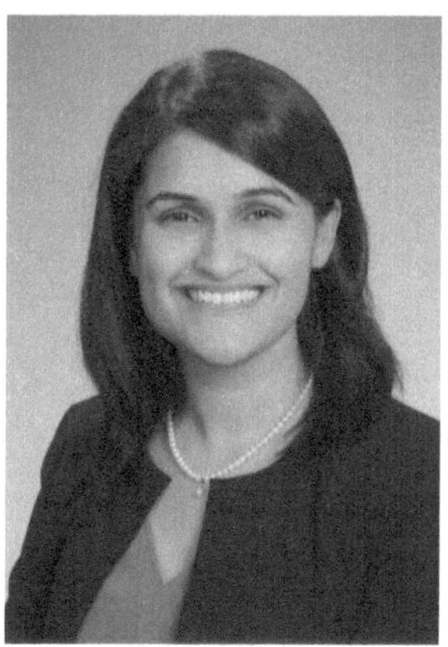

Sampada Deshpande DDS, is a general dentist based in the San Francisco Bay Area. Born and raised in the Middle East, she chose Manipal University to be the beginning of her career in dentistry. She continued her education at the University of Washington, receiving a Doctor of Dental Surgery in 2018. Outside of clinical practice, she teaches coursework at the New Dentist Business Club, stays involved with organized dentistry, serves as Faculty at the University of the Pacific, and advises Samsotech on their IT solutions pertaining to the healthcare industry.

She lives in the city with her husband and can often be spotted riding a bike wearing a *UW dentistry* jersey.

For speaking opportunities, head to sampadadeshpandedds. com for more information. To say hello, you can reach Sampada directly @dr.deshpande on Instagram.